POSTPARTUM MOOD AND ANXIETY DISORDERS

A CLINICIAN'S GUIDE

Cheryl Tatano Beck
DNSc, CNM, FAAN
Professor, University of Connecticut
School of Nursing

Jeanne Watson Driscoll
PhD, APRN, BC
Principal: JWD Associates, Inc.

JONES AND BARTLETT PUBLISHERS
Sudbury, Massachusetts
BOSTON   TORONTO   LONDON   SINGAPORE

World Headquarters

Jones and Bartlett
  Publishers
40 Tall Pine Drive
Sudbury, MA 01776
978-443-5000
info@jbpub.com
www.jbpub.com

Jones and Bartlett
  Publishers Canada
6339 Ormindale Way
Mississauga, ON L5V 1J2
CANADA

Jones and Bartlett
  Publishers International
Barb House, Barb Mews
London W6 7PA
UK

Jones and Bartlett's books and products are available through most bookstores and on-line booksellers. To contact Jones and Bartlett Publishers directly, call 800-832-0034, fax 978-443-8000, or visit our website www.jbpub.com.

Substantial discounts on bulk quantities of Jones and Bartlett's publications are available to corporations, professional associations, and other qualified organizations. For details and specific discount information, contact the special sales department at Jones and Bartlett via the above contact information or send an email to specialsales@jbpub.com.

Production Credits
Acquisitions Editor: Kevin Sullivan
Production Director: Amy Rose
Associate Production Editor: Tracey Chapman
Associate Editor: Amy Sibley
Marketing Manager: Emily Ekle
Manufacturing and Inventory Coordinator: Amy Bacus
Composition: Arlene Apone
Cover Design: Timothy Dziewit
Cover Image: © Photos.com
Printing and Binding: Malloy, Inc.
Cover Printing: Malloy, Inc.

Library of Congress Cataloging-in-Publication Data
Beck, Cheryl Tatano.
 Postpartum mood and anxiety disorders : a clinician's guide / Cheryl Tatano Beck and Jeanne Watson Driscoll.
     p. ; cm.
 Includes bibliographical references and index.
 ISBN 0-7637-1649-9 (pbk.)
 1. Postpartum psychiatric disorders. 2. Postpartum depression. 3. Affective disorders. 4. Anxiety in women. 5. Mothers—Mental health. 6. Childbirth—Psychological aspects. 7. Motherhood—Psychological aspects.
 [DNLM: 1. Depression, Postpartum—diagnosis. 2. Depression, Postpartum—therapy. 3. Anxiety Disorders. 4. Mood Disorders. WQ 500 B393p 2006] I. Driscoll, Jeanne. II. Title.
 RG850.B43 2006
 618.7'6075—dc22

                                                                    2005007809

Printed in the United States of America
09 08 07 06 05   10 9 8 7 6 5 4 3 2 1

To our mothers, Nancy Tatano and Lorraine Watson, without whose love and support we would not be the women we are today.

CONTENTS

FIGURES

TABLES

Chapter 1

Introduction

In 1993, at the annual convention of the Association of Women's Health, Obstetrical, and Neonatal Nursing in Reno, Nevada, we (Cheryl and Jeanne) were walking down the hall from opposite directions when our eyes met each other's name tag; our walking came to a halt. We were finally going to meet, something that each of us had hoped would happen for a long time. We were aware of the other's experience and contributions to women's health. It was the meeting of kindred spirits. It was that meeting that had set the stage for the evolution of the book that you are holding.

Over the years, we have collaborated in various facets of research and education. Using the metaphor of the hand and glove, we have been a perfect fit—the researcher and the clinician. I (Cheryl) invited Jeanne to be a member of my research team in the validation of the Postpartum Depression Screening Scale. As a result of that connection I (Jeanne) enrolled in the doctoral program at the University of Connecticut, with Cheryl as my major advisor. Five years later, with my doctorate behind me, we arrive at this collaboration, *Postpartum Mood and Anxiety Disorders: A Clinician's Guide*. The premise of this book is the integration of research and clinical practice. This partnership of our research program (Cheryl's) and clinical practice (Jeanne's) is the cornerstone of this book. Cheryl brings to this book over 20 years of researching postpartum mood and anxiety disorders. Jeanne brings over 24 years of clinical practice as a psychiatric clinical nurse specialist in private practice focusing on the mental health care of women during their reproductive years. It is the alliance of practice and research that leads to advances in clinical practice, theory development, and policy.

The goal of this book is to provide clinicians with an up-to-date presentation of the mood and anxiety disorders that can occur during the postpartum period. The state of the science of identifying and caring for women with mood and anxiety disorders is evolving. However, few evidence-based treatment models have been published for postpartum disorders. The general theme is that the disorders are similar to those that occur when there is not a pregnancy and a postpartum period; however, most of the research in the care of women with mood and anxiety disorders is derived from the general population studies. Many of the treatment protocols are derived from experience with male and female disorders. Limited data are available regarding the differences in the female and male biochemistry and neurochemistry. The study of sex-specific psychiatry is evolving (Benazzi, 1999; Burt & Stein, 2002; Frank, 2000; Leibenluft, 1999). Postpartum disorders are generally mentioned as a special situation in the studies pertaining to mood and anxiety disorders because the use of medications during the childbearing years is an area of caution and risk management (Altshuler et al., 2002; Hendrick, Altshuler, & Burt, 1996; Legato, 2002).

This book is setting the stage to move the science to the next level. The purpose of this book is not to dictate a singular model of treatment but rather to stimulate creative thinking in the assessment process and treatment plan. We have had the privilege and honor of meeting courageous women who have trusted us by sharing their stories and continuing to reinforce for us that there is no cookbook approach to caring for women who are experiencing mood and anxiety disorders during the postpartum period. The healing relationship involves collaboration, sharing, negotiation, and care. The process of assessment, diagnosis, and treatment involves the development of trust and rapport, a curious mind, and a willingness to think outside of the box. No two women are alike: psychologically, physiologically, culturally, and spiritually. The therapeutic liaison is based on mutuality, reciprocity, and empathic connection (Jordan, Kaplan, Miller, Stiver, & Surrey, 1991; Peplau, 1991).

We have structured the chapters to contain information regarding each diagnosis, treatment suggestions, and a case study using the Earthquake Assessment and NURSE program. Each chapter begins with the DSM-IV diagnostic criteria for that particular disorder and enlarges on its relevance to the postpartum period. We do not provide any cookbook treatment plan because, based on our assumption and years of experience, no such thing exists. Thus, we hope to provide for you a launching place, a place for you to begin to challenge your current knowledge and to listen to women's stories with respect, curiosity, and concern.

In Chapter 2, we present the assessment process using the Earthquake Assessment Model (Sichel & Driscoll, 1999). A general overview of the concept of individual treatment planning via comprehensive assessment and the development of the NURSE program is presented and described. In Chapter 3, the transitory syndrome of the maternity blues is the focus. Our first case studies are presented: maternity blues and complicated baby blues. Chapter 4 presents information on postpartum psychosis beginning with the DSM-IV diagnostic criteria and moving into treatment. The chapter ends with a case study. In Chapter 5, a major depressive episode with postpartum onset takes center stage. This is the area where much of Cheryl's research has occurred. Both her qualitative and quantitative research findings are included in this chapter. Specific sections of this chapter include risk factors, epidemiology, culture, phenomenology, and depression in adolescents, adoptive mothers, pregnancy loss, and fathers. Also addressed are sections on the effects of postpartum depression on children's cognitive and emotional development. Various treatment approaches and a case presentation conclude the chapter.

Chapter 6 presents information on bipolar II disorder (the postpartum depression impostor). Overview, assessment, treatment, and a case study are addressed. Also included are some of the results of Jeanne's doctoral dissertation—a qualitative study concerning the experiences of women living with bipolar II disorder. In Chapter 7, postpartum anxiety disorders are considered. Included in this chapter are panic disorder with a postpartum onset, qualitative data, treatment, and a case study. Obsessive–compulsive disorder with postpartum onset is reviewed with assessment, treatment, and a case study. In Chapter 8, the focus is posttraumatic stress disorder secondary to birth trauma. Some of Cheryl's latest research findings are presented, along with implications and treatment. The chapter ends with a case study. In Chapter 9, screening for postpartum anxiety and mood disorders is highlighted. Various screening instruments are discussed that are useful for the clinician in the assessment process. One of the instruments described is the Postpartum Depression Screening Scale (PDSS), developed by Cheryl and Robert Gable, EdD based on her series of qualitative studies.

The goal, as we stated previously, is to stimulate the ongoing evolution of the specialty area of mental health, psychiatry, and women's health. Women need to be seen, cared for, and their voices heard. The identification and treatment of postpartum mood and anxiety disorders are public health issues in that untreated illness can lead to altered functioning of women as they develop in their maternal role and the development of their infants and family.

References

Altshuler, L. L., Cohen, L. S., Moline, M. L., Kahn, D. A., Carpenter, D., Docherty, J. P., et al. (2002). Expert consensus guidelines for the treatment of depression in women: A new treatment tool. *MentalFitness*, 1(1), 69–83.

Benazzi, F. (1999). Gender differences in bipolar II and unipolar depressed outpatients: A 557-case study. *Annals of Clinical Psychiatry*, 11(2), 55–59.

Burt, V. K., & Stein, K. (2002). Epidemiology of depression throughout the female life cycle. *Journal of Clinical Psychiatry*, 63(Suppl. 7), 9–15.

Frank, E. (Ed.). (2000). *Gender and its effects on psychopathology.* Washington, DC: American Psychiatric Press.

Hendrick, V., Altshuler, L. L., & Burt, V. K. (1996). Course of psychiatric disorders across the menstrual cycle. *Harvard Review of Psychiatry*, 4, 200–207.

Jordan, J. V., Kaplan, A. G., Miller, J. B., Stiver, I. P., & Surrey, J. L. (1991). *Women's growth in connection: Writing from the Stone Center.* New York: Guilford Press.

Legato, M. J. (2002). *Eve's rib: The new science of gender-specific medicine and how it can save your life.* New York: Harmony Books.

Leibenluft, E. (1999). Gender differences in major depressive disorder and bipolar disorder. *CNS Spectrums*, 4(10), 25–33.

Peplau, H. E. (1991). *Interpersonal relations in nursing: A conceptual frame of reference for psychodynamic nursing.* New York: Springer Publishing Company.

Sichel, D., & Driscoll, J. W. (1999). *Women's moods: What every woman must know about the brain, hormones, and emotional health.* New York: William Morrow Publishers.

CHAPTER 2

THE PROCESS OF ASSESSMENT

Postpartum mood and anxiety disorders occur along a continuum from mild to severe. In light of this, the clinicians must collect much data from the woman and her family to ascertain the level of symptomatology and the effect of the symptoms on her daily life. The contexts, the experiences of living with a new baby, in which these disorders occur create in our minds a public health emergency. Mood and anxiety disorders occurring in the postpartum period must be diagnosed and treated as soon as possible because the mother–child relationship, as well as the family development, is at risk.

A critical issue that affects the rates of occurrence of these disorders is the issue of diagnosis. There is no agreed-on time period called "postpartum." The American College of Obstetricians and Gynecologists defines the postpartum experience as the 6 weeks after the birth of a baby. It is thought that at that time the physiologic healing has taken place and the reproductive organs are healed from the pregnancy. A physical examination is done to assess physical recovery and, in essence, to signify the end of the pregnancy/postpartum experience.

The American Psychiatric Association defines postpartum as the first 4 weeks after the birth of a baby. In fact, in the Diagnostic and Statistical Manual of Mental Disorders (American Psychiatric Association, 2000) there is no diagnosis of postpartum depression. The term postpartum is used as an onset specifier, the time when the disorder presents itself. Thus, for example, the diagnosis of a depression that occurs after the birth of a baby is called a major depressive episode with a postpartum onset. This will give you some idea as to why the statistics regarding occurrence rates are not accurate: the statistics depend on how postpartum is defined. In this book, postpartum is defined as the first year after the birth of a baby. For an adoptive mother, it is also the first year after the baby came into her family.

Clinically, it has been our observations that often women suffer in silence for weeks, sometimes months, before they seek help. They live with the hope that the symptoms will go away over time "if I could only get more sleep and more help." Women often blame themselves for the symptoms, and this blame leads to shame and lowered self-esteem, not only as a mother but also as a woman. There is a cost to this delay in securing help, and it is not financial. The emotional cost is overwhelming and often times takes years to repair. The woman has been functioning in a less than normal mode, and this affects her and her baby, family, and friends. The sooner that she is identified, the sooner treatment can be initiated and recovery begun.

The key aspect to a diagnosis of postpartum mood and anxiety disorders is the assessment process. The woman will present with a myriad of symptoms that need to be heard, clarified, validated, categorized, and operationally defined. The assessment process is dynamic and fluid. Women are multidimensional beings and have unique perspectives and/or perceptions of their worldview. As a clinician, the most important aspect of the assessment is to listen to the woman's story. Her story is unique to her and usually does not fit into any "paradigm" or "diagnostic category." You, as the clinician, need to be aware of your own triggers and personal perceptions of mental illness and postpartum occurrences. Be clear and careful that you are not projecting onto the woman any of your own preconceived or premature diagnoses. Each woman's presentation is distinctive to her and her experience. Listen to the words that she uses, and more importantly, listen for the silences, the sighs, and the change in breathing patterns and for the undisclosed. The empathic connection is significant in this assessment. Many women have never gone to a health care provider for issues of emotional and/or mental problems/symptoms. Be alert for the shame, blame, and self-disparaging comments the woman may make about herself and her role as a mother. Be attentive to the nonverbal communication. Gently ask the probing questions while developing the rapport and trust that are essential to the collection of emotional and/or psychiatric assessment information. Remember that assessment is a continual process and is a critical element of every visit.

The assessment process that I (Jeanne) use is based on the Earthquake Assessment Model, published in 1999 by Deborah Sichel and myself in our book *Women's Moods* (Sichel & Driscoll, 1999). This assessment model is based on the geologic phenomenon of earthquakes. Earthquakes occur when the internal pressures on a destabilized subterranean fault line become overwhelmed or pressured. To relieve the internal pressure, the fault line ruptures with great force, and the earthquake occurs. The earth's crust is broken open, and significant chaos and destruction occur above. When the earthquake has settled, the fault line shifts and is vulnerable to pressure of the rocks near it and sits in a state of altered stillness until the pressure builds again. Tremors often occur before the earthquake in response to the pressure on the rocky fault line under the earth's surface. The tremors are felt by the people above and are a reminder that instability exists below.

Sichel and Driscoll (1999) equated the basic brain biochemistry with the fault line beneath the earth's crust. If the surface of the earth above the fault line appears intact, then a woman will present herself as "feeling fine" even if her brain is overloaded and strained. Eventually, the weight of the stressful life events and/or her hormonal events will disrupt the exquisite balance of brain biochemistry, and "an emotional earthquake" will occur (Sichel & Driscoll, 1999). Often women describe "tremors" that have occurred before the emotional earthquake. These tremors may be the onset of mood/anxiety symptoms in response to stressful life events, relational disconnections, or secondary to the use of exogenous hormones. The tremor was bothersome but often did not require medication, although the woman may have sought therapy/counseling to help her with that event in her life. These tremors, however, increase the vulnerability of her fault line and sensitize her to the potential for an earthquake episode. Often, pregnancy and postpartum can be the events that trigger the earthquake. Her outward appearance has changed. Her symptoms are getting in the way of her everyday living; thus, her quality of life is altered, and she often feels that she is "losing" her mind.

The basic structure of the Earthquake Assessment Model (Sichel & Driscoll, 1999) is shown in Figure 2.1. The x-axis is related to the chronological years of a woman's life. The y-axis contains the various biochemical physiologic areas that can be affected by life: life events and responses (stress hormones), reproductive events (reproductive hormones), and the basic biochemical fault line (genetic foundation). The significant events that impact brain biochemistry can then impinge on the external appearance or how the woman's symptoms present.

The assessment process is based on the mapping of the underlying fault lines. The three critical areas of assessment include genetic brain biochemistry, reproductive hormonal biology, and life events or stressors—

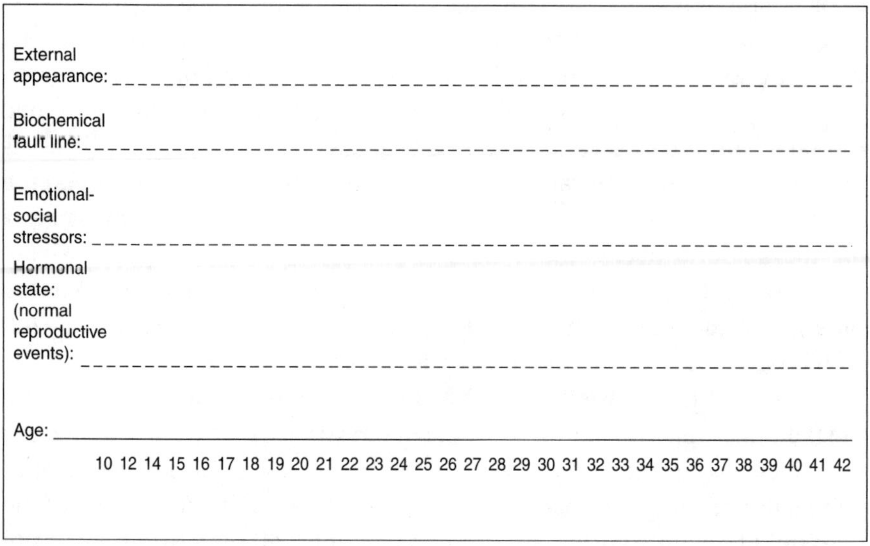

External
appearance: _

Biochemical
fault line: _

Emotional-
social
stressors: _

Hormonal
state:
(normal
reproductive
events): _

Age: _____

10 12 14 15 16 17 18 19 20 21 22 23 24 25 26 27 28 29 30 31 32 33 34 35 36 37 38 39 40 41 42

Figure 2.1 The Earthquake Assessment Chart (Sichel & Driscoll, 1999, p. 100).
Permission is given by Harper Collins Publishers, Inc.

predictable, unpredictable, or traumatic (Sichel & Driscoll, 1999). On the Earthquake Assessment Chart, the top line, the external appearance line, is like the earth's crust, and it covers the gases underneath. As Sichel and Driscoll stated, "A woman's external appearance can reveal little about what is taking place in her brain biochemistry, unless she complains of symptoms that have pushed through the surface" (pp. 100–101). The only way that we can assess whether the brain is in trouble is by the symptoms that the woman exhibits or complains of that are seen as changes in the external-appearance line. That is the line that makes brain strain visible.

Brain strain is the term that Sichel and Driscoll (1999) used to describe the concept of "allostatic loading." Brain strain presents itself through physical ailments such as fatigue, anxiety, headaches, difficulty concentrating, and feeling overwhelmed. It is the brain's way of telling you that it is overloaded. Bruce McEwen (1995, 1998) described allostatic loading as the result of the brain slowly becoming overloaded with stress and the eventual loss of its ability to cope. McEwen defined allostasis as the body's ability to adjust and adapt when it is subjected to increased workload or stressors. The stress response is the body's defense. It is also known as the fight-or-flight reaction or response. This biochemical response helps us to react in an emergency and cope with change. The response triggers the biochemical response needed to arm the body physiologically with what it needs to respond to an emergency: increases heart rate, increases oxygen levels, promotes mental alertness and acuity, and increases the immune response to protect against infection. Thus, when the stress response is chronically activated, it can cause damage to the biochemical systems and the end organs of the hormonal responses and can accelerate disease. The major paradox of the stress response system is that it protects under acute circumstances, but when stimulated chronically, it can damage and hasten disease states. Thus, brain strain, also known as allostatic loading, is visually represented on the Earthquake Assessment Model as changes in the external appearance line.

Now, we will take each assessment domain and focus on the pertinent information that you need to collect in the evaluation and assessment process.

Genetics

Research has shown that there is a genetic link exists in the etiology of mood and anxiety disorders. The basic genetic wiring of each woman was constructed at fertilization of the egg, the DNA of each parent; in fact, the genetic legacy of both families of origin is embedded in the DNA of each person. This genetic hardwiring, in essence, sets the stage for the individualized responses to the impact of events both external and internal on the brain biochemistry. This hardwiring metaphor can be further developed to describe how some systems or circuits can respond to overload and handle it well, whereas other circuitry systems will blow a fuse when the circuit is overloaded. Why can some people respond to significant stressors and have no lasting effects, and for others the stressors cause chronic symptoms?

The first area of information that there needs to be collected has to do with the family history. Most clinicians are very comfortable asking patients about a family history of heart disease, diabetes, and or cancer. The issue of psychiatric family history is often neglected or quickly brushed over. However, as it becomes clear that a genetic link to diseases exists, there is potentially a biochemical etiology for psychiatric illnesses. The critical questions that need to be asked have to do with ascertaining the information about family psychiatric history. When conducting an assessment, the language that is used to ascertain the information is critical to the data that will be obtained. If jargon is used, then the answers will probably be limited and not specific to the uniqueness of the woman, especially if you ask yes or no questions.

Set the stage for an accurate assessment with promoting comfort, establishing rapport, and establishing the foundation for trust and honest disclosure. Sadly, a stigma still exists in the area of psychiatric illness and the cultural marginalization of feeling "out of control" or "losing one's mind." Thus, the setting needs to be established so that the patient feels supported and cared for, not judged or shamed with regard to her feelings and thoughts. Examples of questions are as follows:

- Is there any history in your family of mood and/or anxiety problems/disorders?
- Is there any family history of alcohol and/or substance use/abuse?
- Describe for me what it was like living with your mother, your father, and your siblings. (You are trying to uncover the presentation of mood and/or anxiety problems/disorders in the family, although the persons were never diagnosed. Often women have shared with me that their mother should have been diagnosed, that they have not left their house for years, that there were times when their mother would not talk to them for days and take to her bed, and that their father would come home from work and sit in his chair in front of the television drinking a few beers or cocktails and fall asleep in the chair while their mother would encourage them to speak softly and not disturb Daddy.)
- Did either of your parents demonstrate any extremes of moods? Did you witness times when one or the other had episodes of energy and focus, such as clean the house in a day, paint a few rooms, and decide to rebuild the staircase, and then run out of energy, leaving the project incomplete? (With this question, we are trying to uncover any mood swing episodes of mania and/or hypomania.)
- Was there any history of gambling in your family?
- Did anyone spend a lot of money and then have to return things or deal with debt? (With this question, you are trying to uncover any mania or hypomania history.)
- Was there or is there any time that you felt scared of members of your family? (This question is to attempt to uncover any issues of domestic/family violence.)
- Do you feel scared of anyone in your family now?
- Has anyone in your immediate or extended family attempted suicide or committed suicide? Are there any homicidal events in your family of origin? (A history of suicidality in the family is a high-risk flag for mood and anxiety disorders.)
- Do you remember your mother ever experiencing any mood and/or anxiety disorders around any of her reproductive events? What about

postpartum disorders or issues with menopause—naturally induced or surgically induced?

- Has anyone in your family been on medication to treat mood and/or anxiety problems/disorders, for example, Prozac (fluoxetine), Zoloft (sertraline), Wellbutrin (bupropion), Paxil (paroxetine), Lexapro (escitalopram), and Celexa (citalopram)? Has anyone in your family that you know of ever been taking lithium, Depakote (divalproex sodium), or any other mood-stabilizing agents?
- Is there a history of seizures in your family?

Life Events/Stressors/Responses to Them

The next domain that needs to be assessed pertains to life events or life stressors and the woman's individual responses to those events. Remember that where there is an earthquake, tremors have been taking place, although they may not be felt intensely (i.e., disrupted one's quality of life). For many women, although they have experienced reactions to events, the tremors are often viewed as normal developmental or situational stressors. However, based on the biochemical data, the accumulation of stressors has an impact on the brain biochemistry and can increase vulnerability to mood and/or anxiety disorders at a later stage and phase of one's life (Post, Leverich, Xing, & Weiss, 2001). The assessment process again requires the establishment of rapport and empathic connection during the process. Remember that you will be assessing at every meeting—as the assessment process is continual and as the relationship evolves between the provider and the patient—more and more history is revealed and uncovered. The establishment of trust in the relationship will take time; it is also dependent on the patient's personal history with trust/mistrust issues in relationships.

I use the chronological chart to base the questions in this domain of life events/stressors. I begin by asking the woman whether she has any significant memories from her birth to the age of 5 years. If there is a positive response to this question, the event is placed on the scale, and then the next question pertains to what those memories are: good, bad, and/or traumatic. Were there times when she felt emotional responses to the events: feelings of sadness, isolation, withdrawal, headaches, stomachaches, gastrointestinal disturbances, and so forth?

The assessment process continues moving up the ages and stages of life, documenting any significant events and her response to these events.

As the data collection continues, you may begin to see events that are pushing onto her biochemical fault line. Examples of questions to be asked include the following:

- Were there any significant times in your life when you felt sad or blue, gained or lost weight (without trying), experienced sleep problems— either wanting to sleep all of the time or having no desire to sleep, feeling awake and energized?
- Were there any times that you remember feeling irritated, agitated, easily enraged, or angry?
- Do you drink alcoholic beverages? If yes, how often and how many?
- Were there any times in your life that you had issues with food: anorexia, bulimia, purging, and/or binging behaviors?
- Do you use any substances to alter your mood—heroin, cocaine, marijuana, or Ecstasy? Have you ever used them? Do you remember what your reaction was at the time?
- Were there any times when you were physically, emotionally, or sexually abused? Did anyone ever touch you inappropriately? (If the answer is yes, ask the patient to enlarge on that experience, such as did she tell anyone about the event, and what were the consequences of that.)
- Were you ever in therapy/counseling? If so, for how long? Is that therapist/counselor still around? (If she has a history of a therapy relationship, this will be a source of additional information, or she may want to get back into therapy with that person if she felt that it was a good relationship rather than begin to see a new person in treatment.)
- Have you ever been prescribed medication for anxiety and/or depression? If yes, what medications?

Reproductive Hormonal Events

A woman's reproductive hormonal system is an intricate part of the interconnection of the brain structures, neurochemistry, and stress neurobiology. The menstrual cycle presents an ever-changing hormonal milieu in a woman's biology. The menstrual cycle for most women occurs for greater than 40 years of her life if she lives to about 80 years of age. There are many assessment questions in this domain. This area of a woman's health is often invisible to the normal assessment process in that the assumption is that if no one complains then things must be fine. However, because of the invisibility of the menstrual cycle in the public domain, many women have suppressed, denied, and/or silenced their experiences during their reproductive lives.

The menstrual cycle begins before the onset of bleeding, as it begins with the dialogue between the brain and the ovaries. This premenarche experience can also be a time of the onset of anxiety and/or depression symptoms. The incidence of depression for women compared with men seems to double at puberty or at the time of menarche (Kendler, Thornton, & Prescott, 2001; Kessler, McGonagle, Swartz, Blazer, & Nelson, 1993; Kessler et al., 1994). Many women suffer in silence with the psychologic side effects of oral and/or depot contraceptive agents because depression may be better than pregnancy! Thus, take your time with this assessment domain and listen to the nuances of her experiences. Critical assessment questions for this domain include, but are not limited to, the following:

- When was the onset of your first period?
- Do you remember experiencing any mood or anxiety symptoms before the onset of your first period, such as headaches, diarrhea, stomachaches, anxiety, food issues, cutting behaviors, increased worries, and/or concerns?
- Have you ever been on birth control pills? What was your response to them? Have you ever received a shot for preventing contraception (Depo-Provera), and what was your response, if any, to that?
- Have you ever had an intrauterine device? If so, what type? Did you experience any mood changes after the insertion?
- Have you ever been pregnant? If yes, how many times? (You will be assessing each pregnancy and postpartum experience.)
- Have you ever experienced an abortion or miscarriage? If yes, what was your emotional experience in response to that event? Have you had any counseling/therapy?
- Have you experienced infertility?

  ○ If yes, were you ever given any medications to treat infertility?
  ○ Do you remember what they were and how you felt on them?

- Now we will go through each pregnancy experience and postpartum experience. (Collect information on each pregnancy as a unique experience as well as the postpartum experience. There can be exacerbation of mood/anxiety symptoms during pregnancy and postpartum.)

  ○ Was the pregnancy planned? How long did it take to get pregnant?
  ○ How did you feel during the first trimester? (This is often a time of emotional responses that are often written off easily as "normal" in the first trimester when the body is undergoing the major hormonal assault on the physiologic system. There appears to be about a 10% incidence of undiagnosed depression during the first trimester of

pregnancy; thus, this information is important [Altshuler et al., 2002; Llewellyn, Stowe, & Nemeroff, 1997].)

- ○ What about the second trimester?
- ○ What about the third trimester?
- ○ How did your labor begin? Did it begin naturally, or were you induced?
- ○ Describe the birth experience.
- ○ How did you feel on the first day of the birth? (At this junction, you are assessing the occurrence of any signs of a hypomanic episode that are pertinent in the diagnosis of a bipolar disorder [Sichel & Driscoll, 1999].)
- ○ What was your infant feeding choice: human milk or formula? If you breast fed, how was that experience? When did you wean, under what circumstances, and how was the weaning process experienced? Were there any signs of mood or anxiety symptoms at that time?
- ○ What were the first few weeks like when living with a new baby?
- ○ Did you experience any mood and/or anxiety symptoms during the first year after the birth of the baby? If so, describe this. What did you do about the symptoms?

- Have you ever adopted a child? If yes, do you remember any mood and/or anxiety symptoms that you may have experienced when you took your new baby/child home?
- Please describe your menstrual cycle: regularity, duration, etc.
- Have you ever experienced premenstrual syndrome or premenstrual dysphoric disorder? If yes, please describe symptoms, experience, and any treatment.
- If moving into or are now in the perimenopausal phase of your reproductive life, do you have any symptoms such as irregular menstrual cycles, changes in bleeding patterns, hot flashes/flushes, and night sweats? (A woman can be perimenopausal even if she is still menstruating; it is a process that takes a few years, and thus the changes are erratic and unpredictable. I suggest that women chart their cycles and refer them to the perimenopausal charts in the appendix of the book *Women's Moods* [Sichel & Driscoll, 1999].)
- If you are menopausal, did menopause occur naturally, or was it surgically induced or induced secondary to chemotherapy for cancer?
- Have you ever used hormonal therapy or estrogen therapy?
- Have you ever been diagnosed or treated for a thyroid disorder? If yes, please describe. If you take any thyroid medication, which one and what is the dose?

When collecting the data, you are placing the critical issues on the earthquake chart. You are beginning to get a visual idea of the amount of stressors, through either life events or reproductive events, that have impinged on the brain biochemistry and when tremors or earthquakes have occurred.

Differential Diagnosis

After you have collected the information related to the woman's domains of assessment, the responses are categorized and become the basis for the differential diagnosis of mood and/or anxiety disorders. The assessment is an ongoing process that will be ascertained and updated at each session and/or meeting with the woman. Often, the initial assessment will cause memories and other significant events or experiences to surface; this information will be added to the assessment data.

The key aspects of differential diagnosis are based on the priority issues and/or complaints of the woman. What is getting in the way of her everyday living? Physical symptoms can also manifest with a mood and/or anxiety disorder, and thus it is imperative that those symptoms be included in the assessment data collected (Altshuler et al., 2002; Bellinger, 2000). Somatic symptoms of anxiety can manifest themselves as gastrointestinal symptoms, headaches, chronic pain, shortness of breath, and dizziness (Bellinger, 2000). Thus, the assessment issues of caffeine use, history of thyroid disorders, cardiac arrhythmias, drug use (prescription and over the counter), and possible interactions between medications need to be considered and excluded.

It is important to ascertain when the woman had her last complete physical examination. If it was recently, you will need to get a release to secure this information from her primary care physician, obstetrician, nurse-midwife, and/or nurse practitioner. Question the woman with regard to recent blood tests that have been done and whether she has had any blood tests done recently; if necessary, you will need to secure blood tests. There are the basic blood levels of hemoglobin, hematocrit, white blood cell count, thyroid-stimulating hormone, and T4 that need to be drawn. But if you are thinking that you may be prescribing any atypical neuroleptics or a mood-stabilizing agent, you will need to secure a creatinine, blood urea nitrogen, triglycerides, prolactin, and a blood glucose level as additional data for your baseline data for use with these medications. If your patient has any history of cardiac disorder, you will need to order an electrocardiogram, and if she is presenting with symptoms of anxiety, you may want to talk with the primary care provider/internist to rule out mitral valve prolapse. Remember that you are collecting data that are pertinent to the integration of the biology of the mind and body. The more data you have, the stronger your differential diagnosis can be.

Women's experiences often do not readily fit into any one specific DSM-IV diagnostic category (American Psychiatric Association, 2000). Women often present with symptoms that appear in more than one diagnostic category; thus, based on your own clinical experience, you will be evolving the diagnosis over the visits. However, you will need to pay close attention to the symptoms that are urgent and interfering in her quality of life. If she is not sleeping, that issue needs to be addressed promptly, as the brain will react with major psychiatric symptoms if it is not getting enough time, through deep sleep, to reset and restore itself biochemically and physiologically. When you have come on the diagnosis that you feel her symptoms represent, you need to share that with her, and then describe what that means and how you are going to work with her to help her feel better. It is important to explain that the presentation of these symptoms at this time in a woman's life is not the result of her being a bad person or having a faulty character. I have not met one woman who would choose to have a postpartum mood and anxiety disorder, and I have not met one woman who makes up her symptoms. She is generally so scared and feeling so out of control that our responsibility is to care for her with respect and dignity.

When you have obtained your impressions and/or diagnosis, you will then begin to work with her to design her care plan and to discuss with her how you are going to help her with her symptoms and her healing journey. No specific care plan is available for the treatment of postpartum mood and anxiety disorders. The treatment plans are often based on the expert consensus opinions related to mood and anxiety disorders when a woman is not pregnant, lactating, or postpartum (Altshuler et al., 2002; Hirshfeld et al., 2002).

You must be informed regarding her breastfeeding status, as that will focus your medication choices in the development of your plan. The format for the care plans that I develop with my patients is the NURSE program, which Sichel and Driscoll developed and described in 1999. Over the years, I have found this model to be inclusive and adaptable to updating and changing over the time that I am working with women. I also feel that we need to be living the NURSE program daily as a way to foster and maintain mental and physical health.

The NURSE Program Model of Care

The following section discusses the general care plan developed for a woman experiencing a mood and/or anxiety disorder during the first year after the birth of her baby or the adoption of her baby (Sichel & Driscoll, 1999). The specifics to each disorder are discussed in the chapters that follow as well as a case study presentation using the NURSE program as the format for the care plan.

The NURSE program includes five aspects of care that are necessary to heal from a postpartum mood and/or anxiety disorder: nourishment and needs, understanding, rest and relaxation, spirituality, and exercise. Each aspect is discussed separately and developed in collaboration with the woman. She often can focus on only one or two aspects at a time, but the program evolves to be customized at each stage of her healing. The NURSE program acts as a foundation to build on each aspect a plan that is as unique to each woman as each woman is unique.

Nourishment and Needs

In this section, the areas of focus have to do with food for the body and food for the mind: nutrition, vitamins, fluids, and medications. You will ask the woman what she eats every day and how often she eats. Too often new mothers are not focusing on their own nutrition and needs but rather on their baby and other children, if there are any others. It is necessary to discuss a food plan with her—one that is achievable. She needs to get enough protein every day to heal her body as well as to make milk if she is lactating. We suggest that she eats small meals frequently. We go over protein snacks that are easy to keep in the refrigerator and mobile: cheese, yogurt, turkey, chicken, beef, fish, peanut butter, and so on. Protein drinks are often an easy-to-prepare meal that guarantees that she will get enough protein, too. If you feel that the woman would benefit from a consult with a nutritionist, then refer her. Have a list of referral sources in your own PDA or data files. It is essential that she learn to eat healthy and well. Ascertain whether she is taking any vitamins on a regular basis, and encourage her to finish her prenatal vitamins if she has not, and if she has, then recommend a daily vitamin. Additionally, you will want to assess her calcium intake, as we would like to prevent osteoporosis at a later age and stage of her life. If she does not have a regular intake of calcium-containing foods, recommend a calcium supplement. Some beginning studies have shown that omega-3 fatty acids are helpful in the treatment of depression and mood swing disorders; thus, I recommend the use of fish oil or flaxseed oil to supplement the omega-3s in her diet (Dennis, 2004; Saldeen & Saldeen, 2004; Severus, Ahrens, & Stoll, 1999). The patient should drink at least eight 8-ounce glasses of water per day (especially if she is breastfeeding) and limit her caffeine intake as well as soda/pop/tonic because she does not want to waste her calories on sugary drinks.

Nourishment for the brain includes the use of medications if needed to treat her symptoms. Depending on the diagnostic impression, different medications will be chosen to provide some relief for her symptoms. It is important that the patient is a collaborator in this care plan; thus, you need to discuss with her why you are choosing a certain medication(s), how it will affect her brain, and what the potential side effects are. If she is breastfeeding, be cautious of the medication choices, and provide information to her and her partner regarding the risks and benefits of use of medications with breastfeeding. If she does not want to use medications at this time because of her concerns about breast milk, then discuss therapy with her as well as cognitive strategies and self-help strategies for each facet of her care. If she is comfortable with the information about breastfeeding and medications, then proceed to the prescription process. Specific psychopharmacologic agents are described in the following chapters. Medication choice is part of the art of psychopharmacology because no one specific agent is ideal for any of the disorders that occur during the postpartum period; it is a customized care plan based on symptoms, history, and tolerance.

Needs is the second aspect of this area of the NURSE Program, and in this area you will ask her what she feels that she needs and then negotiate how that can be provided for her. Some women need someone to help them clean, cook, watch the other children if there are any, and so forth. Work with her to find out whether there are any family members or women friends that can come to help her, or whether she and her partner have the financial means to hire some help during this time to reduce some of the pressure.

Understanding

Psychotherapy is, in my opinion, a key element in the treatment of postpartum mood and anxiety disorders. Although medications may be used to treat the biology, the therapy is necessary to treat the psychology. The woman needs to have a place that is accepting, safe, and trusting, where she can talk about how she feels, how the experience has impacted her, and how she is going to grow and integrate the experience. As this is often the first time that a woman has entered into the mental health arena, it is important that she emerges from these disorders in a healthy place and feels empowered in her self and her relationships. As many women have shared with me that they would not wish postpartum illness on their worst enemy. They feel it was in many ways a gift to them because they are able to make sure that they take care of themselves and feel that their recovery and learning has been a gift. Through therapy, they learned more about themselves and their reactions to the world. They were able to move forward with new coping strategies and ways of engaging in interpersonal relationships. They feel more connected in an authentic way. Therapy can be provided on a one-on-one basis or through the use of group therapy models. Support groups specific for women with postpartum illnesses are also very helpful. In my practice, babies are brought to each session. It is a time when I can assess maternal–child attachment and bonding relationships. I can see how the baby is responding to the mother and their face-to-face interactions. Infant development is an important aspect of the therapy because you are helping a woman grow, not only in relationship with herself but also in the relationship with her child. This is another reason why the care of these women is very different than the care of women with mood and anxiety disorders who are not in the postpartum phase of life or are childless.

Journal use is also encouraged as a place to "vomit out" all of the awful feelings that the woman may be experiencing. If she is afraid that someone will read her writings, I encourage her to write them and then burn them in a used coffee can so that she can offer her feelings and thoughts to the gods and goddesses and let them go into the atmosphere. Shredders are also very therapeutic in the destruction of paper that contains personal thoughts, feelings, and/or musings. Privacy and confidentiality are important.

I also recommend books for her and her family to read after she is feeling better. In the early stages of the healing process, she cannot focus enough to read and comprehend the stories. They may also scare her a bit if the women, in their writings, describe personal experiences that are unlike the one that she is having. There is a pervasive fear of getting worse that seems to be evident in many of the women I have met in my clinical practice. A trigger is often if the news media is covering a women who has experienced a postpartum psychosis and there has been an infant death. Postpartum women are highly vulnerable to the news media, both visually and written. Their fear is that they could do something harmful not only to themselves but to their baby. This is why a suicidal and homicidal assessment is done at every contact with the woman.

Rest and Relaxation

Sleep is a necessity for brain care. The brain needs to have deep sleep so that it can restore itself biochemically and physiologically. This is often the area that is first deregulated when a person is experiencing a mood and/or anxiety disorder: They either sleep all of the time or cannot get to sleep, wake early, or have disrupted sleep. The key treatment aspect in this part of the NURSE program is to work with the woman on the development of a sleep hygiene program. She needs to go to bed and wake at a regular time. I have seen clinically that after the sleep patterns are restored, some of the symptoms decrease in severity. A key aspect of helping a patient to get more sleep is the presence of another adult in the home who is willing to help with the night feedings: husband, partner, lover, and/or family member. The goal is to have the woman sleep, a deep sleep, for about 6 to 8 hours for a few nights in a row. Sometimes she feels a lot better after that; at other times, the symptoms are better but not gone. I usually use a small dose of clonazepam (e.g., 0.25–0.5 mg) at bedtime, even if the patient is breast-feeding, and will keep the daily dose of clonazepam to under 1 mg per day (Altshuler et al., 2001; Birnbaum et al., 1999; Saldeen & Saldeen, 2004).

If the patient is breastfeeding, you will have to work with her regarding pumping milk or the use of formula for these night feedings. The care plan has to be customized based on her infant feeding choice.

Periods of rest and relaxation are discussed and planned for in her day. I recommend the use of relaxation breathing (if she had taken childbirth ed- ucation classes she will be familiar with these breathing strategies), yoga, and meditation. I will teach her focused relaxation breathing if she is unfa- miliar with the techniques. We will work together to develop time-saving strategies to use around the house so that she can rest in the day. If possible, the use of family and friends is very helpful in this area of the care plan. Sadly, many women live away from their families of origin when they are starting families; thus, we have to work on creating a new community of care.

Spirituality

In the area of spirituality, the focus is on the experiences of the woman's life that bring her joy, help her to feel uplifted and connected to a power greater than she. It is not defined as organized religion, although if her religion is im- portant to her then that affiliation can indeed fulfill her spiritual needs.

Connected relationships, solitude, appreciation of nature, creative projects, listening to or playing music, gardening and/or keeping a journal are examples of reflective experiences/practices that can nourish the soul.

Belief in God/Goddess or a higher power can also be defined as aspects of spirituality.

The discussion in the process of developing this aspect of the NURSE Program is based on what is important to her and her healing journey.

Exercise

The woman must get exercise because we know that the endorphins that are secreted with exercise can be mood enhancers (Pert, 1997). However, the intensity of the exercise program is based on the number of weeks postpartum. Ideally, if the weather is nice, taking a walk with the baby in the middle of the afternoon is a nice idea. However, if the patient lives in the northern states when it is winter, this is not as easy. After her obstetrician and/or nurse-midwife have given the patient her postpartum checkup, she can begin to incorporate an exercise program. Some women have had a previous regime before pregnancy and are anxious to go back to that. They will, however, have to remind themselves that they have had a baby and need to build up their exercise times and routines. The goal is to have an hour a day of aerobic exercise in her life for the rest of her life, and if we can help her plan and strategize that during this healing process, we are promoting life-long healthy living.

Summary

In this chapter, we have gone over the assessment process and the NURSE program. You have learned that the assessment process is ongoing and that there is not one specific care plan for any of the disorders. The following chapters describe research and treatment strategies for the various mood and anxiety disorders that can occur during the first postpartum year. Each woman is unique, and her story is personal and specific to her genetics, brain biology, and hormones. Listen intently. Consider yourself a detective as you uncover the symptoms and discuss the suggested treatment methods. Work in collaboration with the patient; she is the owner of her experience as well as the person in charge of her healing. I consider my role as a nurse psychotherapist and yours as a clinician involved in the care of postpartum women to be that of a midwife—someone who helps her to grow and develop as a maternal self through the integration of all parts of her authentic self.

References

Altshuler, L. L., Cohen, L. S., Moline, M. L., Kahn, D. A., Carpenter, D., & Docherty, J. P. (2001). Treatment of depression in women 2001. *Postgraduate Medicine Special Report*, 5–28.

Altshuler, L. L., Cohen, L. S., Moline, M. L., Kahn, D. A., Carpenter, D., Docherty, J. P., et al. (2002). Expert consensus guidelines for the treatment of depression in women: A new treatment tool. *MentalFitness*, 1(1), 69–83.

American Psychiatric Association. (2000). *Diagnostic and statistical manual of mental disorders* (4th ed.). Text revision. Washington, DC: Author.

Bellinger, J. C. (2000). Anxiety and depression: Optimizing treatments. *Primary Care Companion Journal of Clinical Psychiatry*, 2(3), 71–79.

Birnbaum, C.S., Cohen, L.S., Bailey, J.W.., Grush, L., Robinson, L. M., & Stowe, Z. N. (1999). Serum concentrations of antidepressants and benzodiazepines in nursing infants: A case series. *Pediatrics*, 104, e11.

Dennis, C.L. (2004). Preventing postpartum depression: Part 1: A review of biological interventions. *Canadian Journal of Psychiatry*, 49, 467–475.

Hirshfeld, R. M. A., Bowden, C. L., Gitlin, M. J., Keck, P. E., Perlis, R. H., et al. (2002). Practice guidelines for the treatment of patients with bipolar disorder. *The American Journal of Psychiatry*, 159(4 Suppl.), 1–50.

Kendler, K. S., Thornton, L. M., & Prescott, C. A. (2001). Gender differences in the rates of exposure to stressful life events and sensitivity to their depressogenic effects. *American Journal of Psychiatry*, 158, 587–593.

Kessler, R. C., McGonagle, K. A., Swartz, M., Blazer, D., & Nelson, C. B. (1993). Sex and depression in the national comorbidity survey I: Lifetime prevalence, chronicity, and recurrence. *Journal of Affective Disorders*, 29, 85–96.

Kessler, R. C., McGonagle, K. A., Zhao, S., Nelson, C. B., Hughes, M., Eshleman, S., et al. (1994). Lifetime and 12-month prevalence of DSM-III-R psychiatric disorders in the United States: Results of the national comorbidity survey. *Archives of General Psychiatry*, 51, 8–19.

Llewellyn, A. M., Stowe, Z. N., & Nemeroff, C. B. (1997). Depression during pregnancy and the puerperium. *Journal of Clinical Psychiatry*, 58(Suppl. 15), 26–32.

McEwen, B. S. (1995). Stressful experience, brain, and emotions: Developmental, genetic, and hormonal influences. In M. S. Gazzaniga (Ed.), *The cognitive neurosciences*. Cambridge, MA: The MIT Press.

McEwen, B.S. (1998). Protective and damaging effects of stress mediators. *The New England Journal of Medicine*, 338, 171–179.

Pert, C. B. (1997). *Molecules of emotion: Why you feel the way you do*. New York: Scribner.

Post, R. M., Leverich, G. S., Xing, G., & Weiss, R. B. (2001). Developmental vulnerabilities to the onset and course of bipolar disorder. *Developmental Psychopathology*, 13(3), 581–598.

Saldeen, P. & Saldeen, T. (2004). Women and omega-3 fatty acids. *Obstetrical and Gynecological Survey*, 59, 722–730.

Severus, W.E., Ahrens, B., & Stoll, A.L. (1999). Omega-3 fatty acids—The missing link? *Archives of General Psychiatry*, 56, 380–381.

Sichel, D., & Driscoll, J. W. (1999). *Women's moods: What every woman must know about the brain, hormones, and emotional health*. New York: William Morrow Publishers.

CHAPTER 3

MATERNITY BLUES

The terms maternity blues, baby blues, and postpartum blues are used to describe a period of time after the birth of a baby when a new mother experiences a myriad of emotions from joy to sadness, organization to confusion, laughing to crying, and confidence to panic. The mood changes come from nowhere, and the mother feels that something is wrong with her. When you think about what has taken place in her body, it is no surprise that the physiologic shift that is taking place causes alterations in her psychologic status as well. The "blues" are usually transitory, and women need reassurance and support. Up to 50% to 75% of new mothers can experience the blues (Miller & Rukstalis, 1999).

The symptoms that women describe include, but are not limited to, sadness, tearfulness, irritability, anxiety, fatigue, worry, and some sleep problems. The blues are basically a normal reaction to the physiologic changes that occur dramatically after the birth of the baby. Generally, baby blues last from a few days to about 3 weeks. A small percentage of women have depression after the blues, especially if there is a prior history of a mood and/or anxiety disorder. A biochemical dysregulation occurs in the brain after the birth of the baby. Estrogen and progesterone, which were at such high levels during the pregnancy, plummet to the lowest levels in such a brief time. This is bound to cause some dysregulation in the brain biology. For many women, however, the brain neurotransmitters and the reproductive hormones reset, and balance is achieved.

In 1952, maternity blues were first described by Moloney as the "third day depression," a mild depression reaction after childbirth. Ten years later, Hamilton (1962) identified this phenomenon as "the transitory syndrome." He interviewed 10 nurses who cared for recently delivered mothers and their infants. The nurses reported that mothers complained of anxiety, fatigue, crying, and confusion.

This self-limited syndrome is generally regarded as a cross-cultural phenomenon. In recent studies, for example, the prevalence of maternity blues has been 65% in the United States (Beck, Reynolds, & Rutowski, 1992), 44% in Hong Kong (Hau & Levy, 2003), 49% in France (Fossey, Papiernik, & Bydlowski, 1997), and 66% in Japan (Nagata et al., 2000). Recently, a lower prevalence rate of 27% was found in Japan with primiparous women who delivered healthy babies by uncomplicated deliveries (Sakumoto, Masamoto, & Kanazawa, 2002).

Recent studies are reporting that the blues peak on the fifth day postpartum, even across cultures. Rohde et al. (1997) discovered in a sample of 86 mothers in Brazil that the blues peaked on the fifth day after the delivery. The peak of the blues symptoms was also on the fifth day postpartum in the United States (Beck et al., 1992) and China (Hau & Levy, 2003).

Maternity blues have been described repeatedly as trivial or fleeting. Evidence is accumulating, however, indicating that across cultures the blues may be a significant predictor of women at risk for developing a depressive disorder later in the postpartum period. In the United States, the severity of maternity blues over the first week after delivery was significantly related to elevated postpartum depressive symptomatology at 6 and 12 weeks postpartum (Beck et al., 1992). In France, a significant relationship was found between the blues at 3 days after delivery and postpartum depressive symptoms 8 months later (Fossey et al., 1997).

Another reason for concern about this seemingly insignificant syndrome has been reported in Japan (Nagata et al., 2003). A significant association was found between maternity blues and weak maternal attachment and elevated anxiety regarding children in mothers between 5 and 10 days postpartum.

Because maternity blues have primarily been viewed as normal in the postpartum period, its clinical significance has not been fully appreciated. The reported prevalence and severity of the blues and their significant relationship to postpartum depression, however, should begin to alert clinicians to the clinical importance of this neglected condition.

In our current health delivery system, new mothers are being discharged early from the hospital, and for many they enter the "dark pit" of postpartum—home alone with no support and/or resources. There is a differential with regard to what is considered normal and what moves into abnormal when it comes to life after baby.

There is a "normal" adjustment period to becoming a mother and, indeed, it is a process rather than an event. This period of childbearing in a woman's life is rarely discussed, leading to feelings of guilt and/or shame that the woman does not match the societal picture of the new mother. Just the physical changes after a birth of a baby can be very different than what the woman expected. She may have had a fantasy that she would have a baby and then go home in her prepregnant clothes, with the reality being that she needs to go home from the hospital in her maternity clothes. She sets up her own expectations regarding her performance, and this is often based on media models or magazine articles. Somehow the truth is easier to face when one thinks about postpartum as a process or transition period.

A lot can be done to help women through this transition to motherhood. Anticipatory education and support regarding what she might expect during the postpartum period need to be provided. The first priority is her physical care. She has experienced labor for hours as well as the delivery process, which may have been vaginal or cesarean, each having its own set of healing issues. Thus, the care of the body and the mind is critical during this early stage of transition. Often the care of the woman experiencing postpartum blues includes normalizing the changes that she is experiencing, the expected trajectory of bodily changes, physiologic and psychomotor skills of lactation, and a real focus on self-care. The major dilemma that many women describe is that there "is not enough time." A sense of chaos and disorder exists. She feels that she never accomplishes a task. The baby is so needy, and she feels insecure and unsure of herself. Often, the mother will describe that in her professional life she was so organized and focused. "What is happening to me now? I don't even know who I am anymore. I feel like I used to get so much done. Now I can't even figure out how to take a shower before 5 p.m.!" The role of the health care provider is one of normalization and support through this transition.

Many of the issues that seem to surface during the early days of the postpartum adjustment have to do with taking on the new role as mother and then the role in the couple relationship as parents. Selma Fraiberg (1956) talked about the "ghosts in the nursery" in relationship to the familial legacies that are present in the parents as they stand around the baby's crib, the history of generations that went before, and how these generations impact on the infant care models of the new parents. For many women who have worked very hard to feel authentic and independent, having a baby puts them into a dependency position, one that requires asking for help. Nevertheless, they assume that they should just know what to do and how to care for a baby. It is a job that requires mentoring and support. Years ago more intergenerational families were living in the same neighborhood, which allowed for more interaction and support for the new mother. Today, many women have been working up to the day of delivery and have no sense of their neighbors or neighborhood.

A tremendous amount of loss is involved in the postpartum process (Driscoll, 1990). A grief process needs to occur so that the woman can mourn the person she used to be and come to accept the person that she is becoming: a mother. The addition of this role to her repertoire of roles can cause some disorganization and disenchantment, phases of transition that have been described by Bridges (1991) in his book *Managing Transitions*.

Bridges defined transition as "the psychological process people go through to come to terms with the new situation" (p. 3). The starting point for a transition is not the outcome but the ending that you have to make to leave the old situation behind. Thus, when a woman moves into post-partum, she has to deal with the ending of the pregnancy and the labor and delivery experience so that she can move into postpartum. This period would be called by Bridges as the "no-man's land" between the old reality and the new. Taking liberty with his phase, we can call "no-woman's land" the time from when she is moving from the role of woman who is pregnant to woman who is mother of a baby. This neutral zone is a time for understanding and gentleness with self. It can be a time of creativity, renewal, and self-development (Bridges, 1991).

The health care provider who cares for women during the postpartum period plays an important role in the provision of support and anticipatory guidance for new mothers as they navigate this transition. A new mother needs to process her experience, mourn the loss of what her fantasy experience had been, and begin to accept what is. Working through the experience is important psychologic work that can be done initially in the early postpartum days by having the woman describe her birth experience and what she had imagined would happen compared with the reality of the experience. You are helping her to debrief, or work through, the events of the experience. Women need to be encouraged to write their thoughts and experiences so that they can do this work. Journal keeping can be a significant adjunctive strategy in addition to verbal discussion and conversation. Helping women to locate and connect with a new mother's support group can be beneficial for many new mothers, as long as the members are honest with their adjustments. Sadly, too many women feel that they must show to the world a "perfect" presentation of their adjustment to motherhood; thus, this does not encourage honest disclosure about how hard it is and the emotional roller coaster that is experienced during this phase of new motherhood.

Case Study: Maternity Blues

Kate is a 30-year-old new mother who phoned and told me that she is afraid that she is losing her mind. She is 5 days postpartum, cannot sleep, and cries "at the drop of a hat." She is terrified that she is going crazy and feels that she needs to be seen immediately. I arrange for her to come to my office the next day. I encourage her to bring her baby so that we can assess their interactions. The next day Kate comes into my office. She looks tired and a bit anxious as she tries to figure out where to put the infant and the infant carrier and seems to be a bit teary as she finds a comfortable spot to sit. She immediately picks up the baby, a little boy, and sits on the couch looking at me. She begins the conversation, "We have worked very hard to get this little baby and now I am wondering why I did this. I don't know what I am doing and I feel like I am a blundering fool. I am so nervous and worried that something will happen to him. I sit all day long holding him and am trying to make him comfortable: trying to breastfeed, changing his diaper (even if he doesn't need it), walking him around, singing to him, and taking walks in the neighborhood. I am exhausted."

My initial goal is to establish rapport with Kate and then to begin to take her history to determine whether she has any risk factors for postpartum mood and anxiety disorders. Based on the assessment data collected, I will then collaborate with her on the development of her care plan, the NURSE program (Sichel & Driscoll, 1999).

The Earthquake Assessment (Sichel & Driscoll, 1999) is based on three sources of information: genetics, life events and personal response to them, and reproductive hormonal experiences. I explain to Kate that I am going to be asking a lot of questions, and that through this assessment we will ascertain, in essence, how her brain got here and how life has dynamically impacted on her brain and its functioning. I explained that postpartum is when many women experience emotional responses, and because of the context of having a new baby to care for, those emotional responses can feel exaggerated and a bit "out of control."

Assessment

Kate described that both of her parents were living and doing well. (Figure 3.1)."They are so excited about this baby. He is their first grand-child." Her parents live about an hour away, and her mom is happy to come and stay with her if she needs the support. She does not remember any history of mood or anxiety disorders. "My mother is pretty calm and laid back. My Dad works a lot but is very helpful to my mom. They get along really well, I think." Kate has one brother who is 5 years younger than her and is currently in medical school in Chicago. "He calls all of the time, and we just sent him pictures of Timmy via the computer." She feels that they had a normal childhood, still has many friends from childhood, and does not feel like she has ever felt like this before. "Jeanne, this is very scary. Am I losing my mind?" I reassured Kate that I really believed that she was experiencing postpartum blues, which is, in many ways, a normal adjustment to motherhood. People do not readily share their feelings—they talk about how great they are feeling and that they are coping well. I continued with the assessment process. "Kate, do you have any memories, good or bad, from the age of birth to 5 years?" She re-

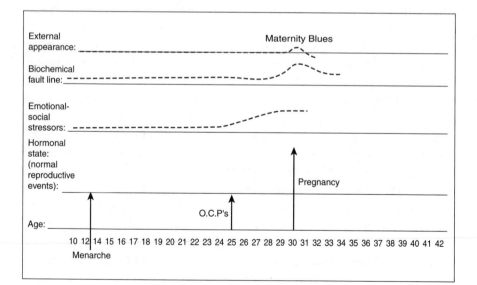

Figure 3.1   The Earthquake Assessment: Kate
Sichel, D. & Driscoll, J.W.: *Women's Moods: What every woman must know about hormones, the brain, and emotional health.* 1999. By permission of HarperCollins Publishers, Inc., p. 100.

membered when her brother was born and how she and her dad went to the hospital. Her dad was on vacation, and she stayed with him. They had a "great time." "We went out to dinner. Afterward, we visited my mom and my baby brother in the hospital, and I helped dad to get things ready for my mom to come home with the baby. I don't remember feeling jealous of him. I remember helping my mom, and also, I had a doll that was my favorite. I still have that doll, and I would imitate my mom. We'd go for walks and all that stuff."

As we moved on to the grammar school years, no significant events had occurred. She described high school as a "good time." She was involved with various activities, sports and musical groups. She had a few boyfriends in high school but no one too special. "I had and have the same best friend from those days. She lives about an hour from us now and is pregnant with her first child, who is due in a few months. I haven't told her how crazy I am feeling because I don't want her to get worried." College was good. She went out of state to college, studied biology, and then got her master's degree in education. "I teach high school biology. I will be going back in September (this was April). I have lots of time to be home and enjoy Timmy, if I ever get to feeling like my old self. (She starts to cry.) This is so scary. I feel so vulnerable and unsure. I've never felt this anxious before."

Kate met Brian in college, and they were married 5 years ago. "He is an electrical engineer and is really excited about the baby. He will be happy to come in here and talk to you. He dropped us off and then was going to park the car and come up here to your office." She described that he is very supportive and "takes good care of me and Timmy, but he is worried. I can see it in his eyes when I am just crying all of the time."

Kate's reproductive history was unremarkable. She experienced menarche when she was 13 and felt prepared for that. "Mom had the talk and all the pads in my closet. In fact, when I got my period, we went out to a girls' lunch to celebrate. I remember that I was never very worried about my period. It came regularly, and I really didn't have any trouble with cramps, headaches, or anything." Kate had taken birth control pills since she was 25 and did not experience any mood changes or any other side effects when she was taking them. She described stopping the pills and having five menstrual cycles before she became pregnant. "We were so excited. We didn't know the sex until he was born. We wanted to be surprised. The pregnancy was uneventful. Although there was some nausea in the first trimester, on the whole, pregnancy was great. I really enjoyed being pregnant. We took childbirth classes and felt really ready for this little guy—but now this." The labor was about 12 hours long. "I pushed for an hour and had no episiotomy and no medication. We were a good team. I was so thrilled to push him out. Brian cut the cord, and Timmy cried right away. He was so tiny and still is (he weighed 6 lbs. 7 oz. at birth and had not been weighed since discharge when he was 5 lb. 15 oz.)." The days in the hospital were okay. "We had a rough start with the breastfeeding, but then he got the hang of it. My milk came in about day 3, when we were home. We went home 2 days after the birth. The breastfeeding seems to be still going okay. He pees and poops regularly. He is fine. It is me. What is wrong with me? My friend Sally, a teaching colleague, told me to call you because you helped her with postpartum depression. Do I have postpartum depression? I don't feel depressed, just sad at times, happy at times, scared most of the time, worried that something will go wrong with him. It doesn't make sense. I know he is healthy. Brian is home with me. He goes back to work next week. Oh that scares me too." Tears are gently streaming from her bright blue eyes. She keeps looking at the baby and kissing his head.

Diagnosis

"Kate, I think you are experiencing the blues and that you are not crazy. You had many expectations of what you would feel like after the baby was born, and what you are feeling right now is normal. When you delivered your baby, the reproductive hormonal levels dropped rapidly from a very high level to a very low level. This rapid change in hormonal levels is thought to cause some reactivity emotionally in new mothers. In addition to those hormonal changes, you are now responsible for this tiny baby that cannot even roll over independently. He is tiny and very dependent. This can be overwhelming at times, especially when you think about your responsibility. Breastfeeding continues that sense of responsibility because you are the nutritional source for your baby. This is a physiologic process, too. Women may experience what feels like hot flashes, sweating episodes, times when they feel confident and joyful, and times when they feel scared and anxious, especially as the baby begins to waken more and makes his or her needs known." I discussed with Kate issues of grief and loss as she begins to mourn who she was before Timmy's birth. The issue of being on call 24 hours per day and having interrupted sleep and nutritional changes can cause many of the symptoms that she is describing. We proceeded to the development of her NURSE program. We invited Brian into the office, shared with him our discussion, and provided him with some anticipatory education and guidance about normal postpartum adjustment issues. Brian appeared very concerned about Kate and shared his thoughts and how he had been trying to help her. He was very attentive and took notes while we went over the NURSE program.

Kate's NURSE Program

N: Nutrition and Needs.

- Meals: We discussed Kate's need to eat small, frequent portions to keep her blood sugar in balance and to have protein at each meal to help with the physical healing of her body and the making of milk. She needed to drink about 8 to 10 glasses of water per day. It would be helpful to fill a pitcher and drink about two full pitchers per day; then she would not have to count every glass. She should continue her prenatal vitamins.

U: Understanding.

- Kate needed to understand the normal physiologic changes that occur after the birth of a baby.
- The use of a journal can be helpful because it allows her a place to purge herself of any worries or concerns and to try to work at letting go. Brian was very open to listening to her feelings, and they shared how they felt very connected emotionally but were just nervous.

R: Rest and Relaxation.

- Sleep is a critical postpartum area of concern. Kate was afraid to sleep because she might miss Timmy's crying and not tend to him promptly. He was sleeping in their bedroom in his bassinet by Kate. She could hear every noise that he made. We discussed putting his bassinet in another room or maybe somewhere else in the bedroom. We also talked about letting him really wake up to eat in the middle of the night so that his feedings would be more vigorous and not just snacks. We also talked about using a relief bottle so that Kate could go to bed early and Brian could keep the baby in the living room while she slept. They wanted a relief bottle but did not want to use formula so soon in Timmy's life. I supported their choice by talking about doing regular pumping to build up a bit of a "milk bank" in her freezer.
- Pumping milk is a learned skill and does require practice and regularity for women to learn to let down to the pump. We discussed the differences between hand-held and electric pumps, and I gave her the proper telephone numbers so that they could obtain a pump.

- We discussed the need for rest periods, as she had just had a baby and her body was very tired from that hard work in addition to the metabolic and fluid changes. She described that her lochia was still bright red and that she did feel very tired. We discussed the expected lochia changes and the issue of physical healing and resting so that the placental site heals well. We spoke about naps, time on the couch, and the need to have Brian care for her while her body healed. I suggested that they take a walk together once a day, and that when Brian went back to work, perhaps they could walk when he got home from work. In fact, when Brian did return to work, would she want her mom to come for a few days to care for them? Often, grandmothers are great sources of support. In addition, they can cook, do laundry, and clean. Kate thought that it would be good to have her parents come. Brian thought that was a good idea so that she would not be afraid to be alone with the baby.

S: Spirituality.

- Kate felt a strong sense of faith that things would get better. She was feeling more relaxed just during this visit. She described to me that she prays to God every day and feels that spiritual connection, "although I don't really go to church regularly."

E: Exercise.

- Because Kate was only 5 days postpartum, there was no rush to begin an exercise program until she had met with her obstetrician/nurse-midwife and had her checkup. Before that, taking walks with the baby in the carriage would be fine, and because the weather was nice, it would be good for her not only as exercise but also as a form of spiritual connection and breathing meditation.
- When she has her checkup, she can resume her exercise program.

The evaluation ended with the plan and an appointment for the next week, because this would help Kate to have a place to talk about her adjustments and her transition into motherhood. We both felt a connection and felt that we could work together. I encouraged her to call me if she had any worries or needed some additional support. I shared with Kate that at this time I did not detect any depression but that we would keep an eye on things. I felt that our meeting for a few sessions would provide the supportive environment that she needed in addition to her partner and her family. She had plans to join a new mothers' group as soon as she felt better and would be collecting more information about various groups in the next few weeks.

After about 6 more weeks, Kate felt more secure in her evolving role as a mother. She felt that she had a sense of Timmy's schedule now and was feeling confident and more secure in herself. We terminated our relationship based on this issue, and she joined a new mothers' group.

Next we discuss a case of complicated blues that required a bit of intervention to help with the postpartum adjustment process.

Case Study: Complicated Baby Blues

It is not uncommon to see a woman who is suffering from what might be called complicated baby blues. The key issue in this diagnostic process is to differentiate between "baby blues" and a major mood and/or anxiety disorder. In my experience, the evaluation process and the relational connection are critical, as the assessment process is ongoing and cumulative. Let us look at a case of a woman who came into my office and discuss the care plan and rationale.

Ginny called my office and left a message. Her nurse-midwife told her to call because she feels as though she is losing her mind and jumping out of her skin. When I returned the call, I learned more about Ginny. It is 2 weeks postpartum after the birth of her son, Evan, and she just feels like she is jumpy and anxious. She describes that she cannot sleep, worries all of the time about Evan, and is breastfeeding. This has been "a challenge and a struggle. I don't know what to do. This is not what I expected would happen. We were ready to have a baby. I feel so scared all of the time. Can you help me?"

We arranged to meet the next day at my office and I encouraged her to bring the baby and her partner with her so that we could all discuss and collaborate on a plan to help her with this experience. The next day Ginny, baby Evan, and her husband, Ron, came to my office. Ron was holding the baby in a car seat/infant carrier. Ginny looked exhausted, red eyed (like she had been crying), and a bit hesitant when I addressed her and introduced myself formally. I asked Ginny whether she wanted to come in alone or if she wanted to bring Ron into my office. "He can come. I have no secrets from him. We are in this together." They all came into my office. As they got settled on the couch in my office, Ron took Evan out of the infant seat and held him in his arms. Ginny just looked at the two of them and then at me; tears were gently streaming down her face. "Can you help me?" she asked.

I explained to the couple that I was going to be asking many questions to ascertain what was going on and what her symptoms were, and then I explained a bit about my assessment process and how it was based on three parameters: genetic history, life events/responses, and reproductive hormonal events and responses. The impact of life on the brain biology influences the symptoms that are presented. The brain will emit symptoms that we need to pay attention to, because the brain is the cornerstone of a woman's mental health. I also usually ask what it was like for her to call a psychiatric care provider in response to her symptoms, and I give some information about my professional history and experience. I feel that that relational connection can help to relax the process of collecting the mental health data and information.

I explained to Ginny and Ron that I was going to try to assess and make clinical impressions about Ginny using her symptoms and history. We would then collaborate on a care plan and discuss follow-up plans. I also encouraged Ginny to feed her baby if she wanted. I was comfortable with breastfeeding, having been a lactation consultant. It is important that women are comfortable breastfeeding in my office because I can ascertain feeding positions, adjust them if needed, and see the maternal infant attachment process. This also applies to women who formula feed their infants in my office. You can really learn a lot by watching how mothers hold their babies and the bottle. You can see whether they are responsive to the babies.

I explained to Ginny and Ron that I was going to begin collecting information about her genetic/family history, about her life and the impact of events on her life, and, finally, her reproductive history and response to those events (Figure 3.2). I began by asking Ginny about her mother. "Ginny, you lived with your mother. Would you describe that she had any mood and/or anxiety disorders? Is she currently alive? How old is she? Does she have any medical problems/conditions? Alcohol use/abuse? What about her mother's mother/father, do they have any mood and/or anxiety disorders/medical problems?" We then discussed her father and his family of origin. In response to my assessment questions, I learned that Ginny thought that her mother was an "anxious mess. She worries about everything and has been calling me two to five times a day asking me how I am doing. She is coming to stay next week. I am not looking forward to that, especially if I feel this way. Her anxiety will push me over." Her mother has never been treated for an anxiety disorder, but she did have a history of atrial fibrillation and flutter, was on Coumadin, and was regularly followed for that condition. Her mother was 55 years old and basically healthy. She was a teacher who was still working, and although she was thinking about retirement, she was not really in a hurry to do that. Her alcohol intake was very rare. She possibly had a cocktail when she went out to dinner but did not drink at home unless they had company. Her father was retired from his job as an engineer and was happy being at home. He had many hobbies and played tennis regularly with his buddies. She did not think that he had any psychiatric problems. He did travel when he was working and was not always available. "He left most of the childrearing to my mother. He would support her decisions, and they seem to be a good pair. They seem to get along really well." She could not remember whether any of her aunts or uncles had any history of mood and/or anxiety disorders.

Ginny was 26 years old and had four siblings: two brothers and two sisters. She was the middle child in the grouping of five. She had an older brother and sister and a younger brother and sister. Her siblings' ages ranged from 24 to 34 years old. Her older brother, Chris, was 34 and married with three children. He did not seem to have any mood or anxiety disorders. "He is a college professor and seems to have a good

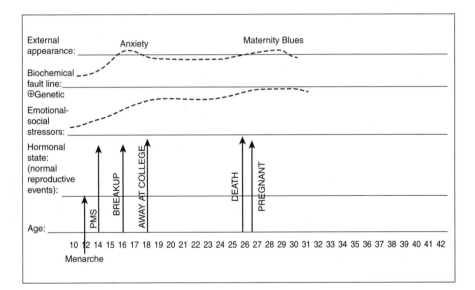

Figure 3.2 The Earthquake Assessment: Ginny
Sichel, D. & Driscoll, J.W.: *Women's Moods: What every woman must know about hormones, the brain, and emotional health.* 1999. By permission of HarperCollins Publishers, Inc., p. 100.

relationship with his wife and children." Her older sister, Liz, was 32 years old and did not have any children. She was gay and lived with her partner for the past 10 years. "I really like her partner, Stacey, and she is such a big help to me. I am closest to Liz; sadly, she lives in another state but is calling me and is so supportive. She has some anxiety and told me that she has been taking Zoloft (sertraline) for years because she had bad premenstrual symptoms of anxiety and irritation. Then there is Michael, who is 29. We are close in years but not close as siblings. He lives in Alaska. He wanted to move far away. He does not get along with my parents at all. He feels that they are controlling and just wanted to get away, and he did. I hear from him mostly through e-mail. Finally, my baby sister, Michaela, who is 24 years old, lives with her boyfriend David. They do not have any children. They both work downtown. She is a mechanical engineer, and David is a lawyer. They met in graduate school and seem to have a good relationship. She is concerned about me and has brought over meals for Ron and me. She loves Evan." At that moment, Ginny looked at me through glistening tear-filled eyes and implored, "Am I going to be all right? I am so scared. I am afraid I am losing my mind and will never find it again. This is such a terrifying experience." I reassured Ginny that she was going to be fine, that I was glad that she had called, and that I was going to take care of her and her family.

We moved to life event assessment and how those events impacted her (good and/or bad). Remember that the purpose of collecting the data in the three domains is to ascertain "allostatic load" or "brain strain" (McEwen, 1995; Sichel & Driscoll, 1999). I asked Ginny whether she could remember any significant events between the ages of birth and 5 years. "Nothing significant. My younger siblings were born, but I do not remember that as being too bad. My grandmother (maternal mother) stayed with us and helped my mom. I really loved my grandmother. She died a few months ago. It was so sad. I really miss her." This was an important piece of information. I would need more information about it as we moved in the data collection. I responded, "Ginny I am so sorry about your grandmother. She died during your pregnancy?" Ginny responded, "Yes, she died of pancreatic cancer. She died within 6 weeks of being diagnosed. She had hospice, and my mom and sibs really did a great job. They were all with her when she died. I was there, too, as was Ron. I think if you have to die, she had a nice death. We all got to say good-bye. I am just so sad that she is not here to meet Evan, and she would have been a big help to me, too." This is a bit of a red flag. Her grandmother's death probably led to a grief reaction and mourning process. We would have to get back to this as part of the evolving care plan.

We then moved to the ages of 5 to 10. Ginny did not remember any significant good or bad events during those years. She attended a Catholic school, had lots of friends in the neighborhood, and could not recall anything noteworthy. We then moved to the ages of 11 to 13 years, puberty. She continued in the same Catholic school until she graduated from eighth grade. "I played soccer in the fall and spring. My dad was the coach. We had a good time." I then asked her about high school and any events. "Well in high school, I had my heart broken by my first boyfriend. It was horrible. Looking back at that I wonder what I saw in him anyway (as she looks at Ron and smiles warmly), but he broke my heart." I asked her to expand on what she meant regarding her broken heart. She replied, "Oh I was devastated. I was a sophomore, and he was a junior. We had been going steady for almost a year, and then I found him kissing another girl at a party at a friend's house. I was so shocked, and then when I confronted him, he told me that I was too controlling and that he did not want to go out with me any more. It was just a sudden break. Then my girlfriend told me that she had seen him with that other girl many times, but she did not want to tell me because she knew that would hurt me." She then proceeded to describe the situation. "I cried a lot and was very sad; my heart was broken. How could he do that to me? My mother was supportive. Of course, he was a jerk in her eyes because he treated her daughter poorly. She was angry. For me, however, I moped about for about a month or so, and then I realized that I had to snap out of it and move on. I did not want him to be that important. I went out with friends and started to heal and have a good time. I was in the theatrical productions and had a lot of friends, many of whom were boys." I gently at one point in the assessment asked whether she had experienced any sexual abuse, inappropriate sexual behavior, and emotional and/or physical abuse. She denied any.

On the whole, high school was not a big thing. "It was normal stuff—no big things. I was ready to go to college." She went to college in another state and had severe homesickness. She had a very difficult first semester at college and missed her family and all of her friends. "I was so homesick. I cried a lot. I called my mom and dad all of the time and lost about 10 pounds. It was a big adjustment, but after about 2 months, I started to connect with people. I got involved in the theater group and some other clubs on campus. That helped, and then I really liked college and did not really want to go home. Weird isn't it?" This was a tremor according to my earthquake assessment model; she had symptoms of anxiety and homesickness and lost weight; she cried, sought support, and came through the experience, but what was the impact on her neuro-transmitters? Again, these data would be integrated into the formulation at the end of the assessment.

She went on to graduate school, where she met Ron. They fell in love, lived together for a few years, and got married 2 years ago. They had planned this pregnancy and had been looking forward to having a baby in their lives. We moved to the reproductive history.

Ginny described that she had started her period when she was about 12 years old. Her mother and her sister helped her prepare for it; thus, it was not a scary event. She was regular and had slight cramps, although she did describe that she would feel a bit anxious before her period and also would drop things easily. "I could always tell that it was coming because I would worry more, and it seemed as though my ability to hold onto things was changed. After my period began, I felt better and would basically forget about the symptoms until my next pre-period time." These symptoms of increased worry premenstrually were a red flag item that would be pursued later in the assessment process. She described that she had used oral contraceptives without any significant side effects.

Ginny had experienced only one pregnancy—this one. She had not taken the oral contraceptives for about 6 months before conception. My aim was to have her now describe her pregnancy and her postpartum experience to date. "I was so excited to be pregnant. Ron was thrilled. Weren't you honey?" She looked at him, and he smiled and nodded. "I was a bit nauseous and did have some vomiting, but it wasn't that bad when I look back on it. I was just glad to be pregnant." She described that her first trimester was uneventful. She did have an amniocentesis at about 16 weeks gestation. "But we didn't want to know the sex. We wanted to be surprised." Her second trimester was a bit different because a big project was due at work and had a deadline. She was working 12-hour days and not sleeping very well. The project ended about 2 weeks before she went into labor. "I was exhausted and yet knew that I had to get the project off my desk so that I could have a nice maternity leave, but I think I am still tired. I was anxious then. Now that I think about it, I was worried that people would not do their jobs even though I work with a great team. My anxiety was a bit over the edge at times. Do you remember, Ron?" Ron looked at her and then at me and said, "She was off the wall, if I can speak honestly. She would worry, obsess, and talk about what had to be done all of the time, and I could not wait for the damn project to be finished. I would encourage her to go to the gym, take a swim, or take a walk, but she was focused and almost mean at times when I was not being supportive. I put in long hours, too, but I know that exercise really helps me. She was a worried mess, and then she transferred the worry after the project was completed into worry about when labor would start. She wanted to stay home nearly all of the time. She would go to work. The project was over; thus, she would be home early, like 5:30 or so, and we would eat dinner together. She was going to bed early, but then in bed, she would move into the "what if" mode. Fortunately, the birth was normal. She had a vaginal birth, and everything was okay—now this. She is falling apart again. I hope you can help us."

I smiled warmly at him and quietly said that I would indeed help them and that we would work together to do it. Through their body language and tone of voice, I felt like they were relaxing more with me. We moved to the most recent history to collect the story of the past few weeks.

"So, Ginny, you shared with me that you worked on the project until a few weeks before the birth. Now tell me what happened after the project was complete up until today." She looked at me, sat back, looked at Evan who was in Ron's arms, smiled softly, and began to talk. She described that she felt exhausted after the project was finished and that she had just figured that everything would go back to normal now that the deadline was met and the project was approved. She thought that would be a great way to go away for maternity leave. She spent those few weeks until she went into labor organizing her office space and giving reports to the colleagues who would be covering for her. "Usually, after I have the project complete, I collapse, get sleep, and after a few days feel less stressed and less obsessive. I don't seem to worry as much, but this didn't happen this time. I couldn't get comfortable in any sleeping position. The baby was low, and I had to go the bathroom frequently. My back hurt. I was a mess. I would cry if Ron looked at me funny. I was eating all right and drinking fluids. I did not feel any pressure at work or home, but I couldn't relax. I walked and talked to my family and friends. My sister-in-law told me that she was always anxious before the birth of all of her children. The birth was really coming, and the worry about whether everything would be okay soaks into your consciousness. I just figured that I'd tough it out, and it would all go away. She said, 'Wait until you see that little baby. You will fall in love and everything will be fine.' She had three babies, so I trusted her and her experience. What a jerk I was!"

She continued to describe the weeks that led up to the birth. They had taken childbirth classes through the hospital but didn't really practice very much. "I did, however, try to do the breathing to calm my anxiety," she said. She began to have contractions on a Tuesday morning. "I guess they were coming about every 15 minutes when I realized what they were. I was 39 weeks pregnant and had seen the nurse-midwife the day before. She said that my cervix was thin and that I was a fingertip dilated, but that that didn't mean that anything would be happening quickly. When I realized that there was some regularity that morning, I called her." She went on to describe how she called the nurse-midwife who answered her questions. They decided that she was in early labor. There was no need to come to the hospital. She should call back when the contractions were about 5 minutes apart. She was encouraged to eat lightly and keep her fluid levels up. She told me that Ron had gone to work. She wanted to call him, but at the same time, she had felt that she got so anxious about everything that she didn't want to worry him if it was going to be a long wait. Thus, she called her older sister. She reassured me and called me back throughout the day until Ron came home. "When he got home, it was about 6 p.m., and the contractions were about 10 minutes apart. They were uncomfortable, but I was walking and talking. He was surprised when he walked in and I told him that we would probably have our baby in a few hours." Ron then jumped into the conversation. "I couldn't believe that she didn't call me. After I got over that, I realized that she was okay and that in a funny way she was much calmer and seemed like the ol' Ginny." Ginny looked at Ron, took his hand, and smiled through her tears.

The birth story continued. The contractions increased in frequency and intensity, and she found that she was getting anxious again and wanted to talk to her nurse-midwife. Thus, they called the nurse-midwife. When she called back, after the assessment, she told them to come to the hospital, and she would see them there. Now the two of them spoke about how they spent a while trying to pull together the suitcase, books, radio, phone list—all of the stuff that they had prepared—but now they both described feeling a bit anxious and disoriented. They finally got in the car. The contractions were about 4 to 5 minutes apart, and they were breathing through the contractions in the car. It took about 35 minutes to get to the hospital. "Luckily it wasn't rush hour, so we didn't hit any traffic," remarked Ron. They arrived at the hospital at 10:00 p.m. They were taken to the labor and delivery suites and admitted.

After vaginal examination, Ginny was about 6 centimeters, and the contractions were intense. She had planned to have an unmedicated birth and was trying to stick with that plan as best she could. The nurse stayed by her side, and "with Ron and the nurse, her name was Carol, I really felt cared for and supported. The transition phase was brutal but I keep focused and was in many ways excited even though I was scared." At 1:00 a.m., she was fully dilated and ready to push. "Boy was I ready. That felt great. It was an amazing feeling of strength to push him out." She described essentially a short second stage of labor of about 1 hour of pushing, and then Evan was born. She did have a tiny vaginal tear but no episiotomy. "When I saw him come out, I just started to sob. I couldn't stop myself," said Ginny. Ron now put his free arm around her and held her close to him. Evan being in his other arm started to stir. I smiled and said aloud, "I think Evan is remembering that too. Look at his little smile." That was a very soft, gentle moment as we all celebrated Evan's birth.

I then encouraged Ginny to continue her story of those next 24 hours and her emotional responses. These descriptors are important pieces that are necessary to fit into the puzzle of the formulation of diagnosis and holistic care plan, the NURSE program (Sichel & Driscoll, 1999).

Ginny described the first day as uneventful. Her family came to visit, and she describes being excited and happy. "The breastfeeding didn't happen as naturally as I had imagined, but we kept persisting. Finally, we both got the hang of that. My nipples are still a bit sore but seem to be getting better." She described that she went to the classes in the hospital and felt that she was doing well until they got home. "My mind began to take over now. I was worried about everything. Was he going to wake up to eat? Would I have enough milk? Was I drinking enough?" Ron described that nothing he did would relax her. He felt that she was doing everything just fine and that the baby seemed fine: sleeping, peeing, and moving his bowels. He felt that she just could not relax.

Ginny then said, "I would get in bed at a reasonable hour, and then I would wait. In fact, I still wait for him to wake up. I am afraid that I won't hear him. I hear Ron snoring, and I am irritated at him. How can he sleep? I am not a very nice person to be around. I am irritable, cranky, and not very nice." Ginny had not had any episodes of deep sleep since the baby was born. She could not nap and felt that she was just becoming "a basket case." She was hard to reassure and seemed to be holding life together with dental floss. I knew that we had to dampen her biology, as the anxiety was pervasive and she felt that she could not get it under control. Ginny had a history of anxiety as well as some depressive episodes. It must have been hard having her much loved grandmother die during her pregnancy, too. I felt that our initial goal should be to help her get a few nights of deep sleep so that we could give her brain a chance to restore itself and recover from the past few weeks of limited deep sleep periods. She was having a somewhat complicated case of the baby blues, and we would help the brain with some medication to help her sleep. Then we could reassess in a few days. We began to collaborate on her NURSE program. Ginny and Ron were told that this plan would be changed regularly based on how she was feeling. We would be essentially focusing on one aspect at a time—in her case, the R section, rest and relaxation. Ginny's initial NURSE program included the following:

N: Nourishment and Needs: Ron reassured me that he was home for the next 2 weeks and that he would make sure that Ginny ate regularly with attention to the proteins and fluids. I suggested that frequent, small meals were sometimes better for maintenance of balanced blood sugars rather than three big meals per day. Ginny would continue her prenatal vitamins and limit her caffeine and chocolate intake.

U: Understanding: They both knew that they could call me with any questions and that we would be touching base for a short time every day for the next few days. The healing process is helped along if the patient feels extra support.

R: Rest and relaxation: This area needed the most attention at this time. I discussed with Ginny and Ron the use of a long-acting benzodiazepine, Klonopin (clonazepam), to decrease her anxiety and to help her sleep. Most of the women that I treat have limited exposure to antianxiety medications; thus, the low doses seem to work adequately and rapidly. I suggested that she take 0.5 mg. of Klonopin at bedtime, which should be at about 9:00 p.m. She was to go to bed, and Ron would be in charge of the baby. We discussed the use of formula even though she was breastfeeding. Although I typically do not like to use formula in the diet of a breastfed baby until about 3 weeks postpartum, I felt that we needed to get Ginny some deep sleep at this time. This would help to reset her brain biochemistry. In a few days, when she felt better, she could resume the night breastfeeding and, in my experience, not lose any milk in the process. Interestingly, after getting more sleep and decreasing the anxiety, she may even find that her milk supply improves as a result of the healing process. We would do this plan for 2 to 4 nights and then reassess how she felt every day.

I wanted her to take 0.25mg. of Klonopin when she woke in the morning and then again around 3 to 4 p.m. I felt that that dose should help her anxiety levels go down and allow her to relax and get in touch with her own coping strategies.

S: Spirituality: We did not get into this area on this visit.

E: Exercise: At this visit, we were not going to address this area until Ginny felt better and her sleep was adequate.

Ron, Ginny, and Evan left my office. The next day I called the house. Ron answered the phone. He said that the baby had taken the bottle of formula from him just fine and that Ginny had gone to bed at about 8:30 p.m. and slept until about 6:00 a.m. He and Evan slept in the living room so that Ginny would not be disturbed. He felt that she was looking better already. His report was encouraging, and then I spoke with Ginny. "I feel like a new woman. I cannot believe how deep I slept. Will that happen again tonight? How long do we do this?" I shared with Ginny that I was happy that she had slept so deeply and asked her how she was doing on 0.25 mg. of Klonopin. She told me that she just did not feel as nervous and that she and Ron were having a nice day so far. The baby was doing well. She was nursing regularly, and she thought that things were much better. We discussed repeating the sleeping plan for that night and agreed to check in again tomorrow.

The next day I spoke with Ginny. She had another good night and felt that she was ready to take back the night feeding. I suggested that she lower the night dose of Klonopin from 0.5 mg. to 0.25 mg. and see how the night went. If she was able to get back to sleep after she fed Evan, that would be a good sign. She told me that she and Ron were optimistic that things were looking up. "Jeanne, I just feel so much better."

She took back the night feeding and was able to get back to sleep after Evan nursed. When they came to my office for the next scheduled visit, she looked so much better and more rested, and her eyes were bright and shiny. We talked about her potential genetic vulnerability to anxiety secondary to how she described her mother as well as the premenstrual anxiety episodes that she spoke about. We discussed normal infant development issues, parenting concerns, and other anticipatory guidance regarding the next few weeks postpartum. We scheduled a meeting for 2 weeks from that day to reevaluate the healing journey.

Ginny, Ron, and Evan did well, and we terminated visits after 2 months. Ginny was to call me if she felt that her symptoms were exacerbating or if she just felt that she needed some therapy in the future. By helping to quiet her brain biology via deep sleep, her brain did some restorative healing, and her usual coping strategies could take place as she learned to be a mother. My hope was also that she had had a positive experience with a psychiatric nurse care provider. Thus, if she did feel that her emotional symptoms were getting in the way of her everyday life, she would not be afraid to call and get some help.

References

Beck, C. T., Reynolds, M. A., & Rutowski, P. (1992). Maternity blues and postpartum depression. *Journal of Obstetric, Gynecologic and Neonatal Nursing*, 21, 287–293.

Bridges, W. (1991). *Managing transitions*. Reading, MA: Addison-Wesley Publishing.

Driscoll, J.W. (1990). Maternal parenthood and the grief process. *Journal of Perinatal and Neonatal Nursing*, 4, 1–9.

Fossey, L., Papiernik, F., & Bydlowski, M. (1997). Postpartum blues: A clinical syndrome and predictor of postnatal depression. *Journal of Psychosomatic Obstetrics and Gynecology*, 18, 17–21.

Fraiberg, S. (1956). *The magic years*. New York: Fireside.

Hamilton, J.A. (1962). *The transitory syndrome*: In *Postpartum Psychiatric Problems* (pp. 107–111). St. Louis: CV Mosby.

Hau, F. W. L., & Levy , V. A. (2003). The maternity blues and Hong Kong Chinese women: An exploratory study. *Journal of Affective Disorders*, 75, 197–203.

McEwen, B. S. (1995). Stressful experience, brain, and emotions: Developmental, genetic, and hormonal influences. In M. S. Gazzaniga (Ed.), *The cognitive neurosciences*. Cambridge, MA: The MIT Press.

Miller, L. J., & Rukstalis, M. (1999). Beyond the "blues": Hypotheses about postpartum reactivity (pp. 3–19). In L. J. Miller (Ed.), *Postpartum mood disorders*. Washington, DC: American Psychiatric Press.

Moloney, J. (1952). Postpartum depression or third day depression following childbirth. *New Orleans Child and Parent Digest*, 6, 20–32.

Nagata, M., Nagai, Y., Sobajima, H., Ando, T., Nishide, Y., & Honjo, S. (2000). Maternity blues and attachment to children in mothers of full-term normal infants. *Acta Psychiatrica Scandinavica*, 101, 209–217.

Rohde, L. A., Busnello, E., Wolf, A., Zomer, A., Shansis, F., Martins, S., & Tramontina, S. (1997). Maternity blues in Brazilian women. *Acta Psychiatrica Scandinavica*, 95, 231–235.

Sakumoto, K., Masamoto, H., & Kanazawa, K. (2002). Postpartum maternity blues as a reflection of newborn care in Japan. *International Journal of Gynecology and Obstetrics*, 78, 25–30.

Sichel, D. A., & Driscoll, J. W. (1999). *Women's moods: What every woman must know about the hormones, the brain, and emotional health*. New York: William Morrow Publishers.

CHAPTER 4

POSTPARTUM PSYCHOSIS

Diagnostic Criteria for Brief Psychotic Disorder

A. Presence of one (or more) of the following symptoms:
   1. Delusions
   2. Hallucinations
   3. Disorganized speech (e.g., frequent derailment or incoherence)
   4. Grossly disorganized or catatonic behavior (do not include the symptom if it is a culturally sanctioned response pattern)
B. The duration of an episode of the disturbance is at least 1 day but less than 1 month, with eventual full return to a premorbid level of functioning.
C. Disturbance is not better accounted for by a mood disorder with psychotic features, schizoaffective disorder, or schizophrenia and is not due to the direct physiologic effects of a substance (e.g., a drug of abuse, a medication) or a general medical condition.

Specify if:

With marked stressor(s) (brief reactive psychosis): if symptoms occur shortly after and apparently in response to events that, singly or together, would be markedly stressful to almost anyone in similar circumstances in the person's culture.

Without marked stressor(s): if psychotic symptoms do not occur shortly after or are not apparently in response to events that, singly or together, would be markedly stressful to almost anyone in similar circumstances in the person's culture.

With postpartum onset: if onset within 4 weeks postpartum (APA, 2000, p. 332).

Major depressive episode with psychotic features:

Severe with psychotic features: This specifier indicates the presence of either delusions or hallucinations (typically auditory) during the current episode. Most commonly, the content of the delusions or hallucinations is consistent with the depressive themes. Such mood-congruent psychotic features include the delusions of guilt (e.g., of being responsible for illness in a loved one), delusions of deserved punishment (e.g., of being punished because of a moral transgression or some personal inadequacy), nihilistic delusions (e.g., of cancer of one's body "rotting away"), or delusions of poverty (e.g., being bankrupt). Hallucinations, when present, are usually transient and not elaborate and may involve voices that berate the person for shortcomings or sins. Less commonly, the content of the hallucination or delusions has no apparent relationship to the depressive themes. Such mood-incongruent psychotic features include persecutory delusions (without depressive themes that the individual deserves to be persecuted), delusions of thought insertion (i.e., one's thoughts are not one's own), delusions of thought broadcasting (i.e., one's actions are under outside control). These features are associated with a poorer prognosis. The clinician can indicate the nature of the psychotic features by specifying with mood-congruent features or with mood-incongruent features (APA, 2000, p. 412).

Postpartum psychosis (PPP) is the most serious and severe form of postpartum mood disorders with high rates of suicide and infanticide (Appleby, Mortensen, & Faragher, 1998). Luckily, it is a rare disorder that occurs in 1 to 2 per 1,000 deliveries (Kendell, Chalmers, & Platz, 1987). Psychosis appears suddenly after delivery, within a few days, and in most cases within the first 3 weeks (Brockington et al., 1981). The majority of these psychoses are either due to bipolar disorder or major depression with psychotic features. The onset is infrequently caused by reactive psychosis or schizophrenia (McGorry & Connell, 1990).

PPP is characterized by symptoms of extreme agitation, confusion, exhilaration, and an inability to sleep or eat. It may be hard to maintain a coherent conversation with a woman who has PPP. She may also experience delusions, hallucinations, an altered and/or impaired concept of reality, rapid mood swings, insomnia, and abnormal or obsessive thoughts. The onset of this disorder represents a psychiatric emergency and warrants hospitalization. It is estimated that up to 5% of women with PPP may commit suicide and that 2% to 4% are at considerable risk of harming their infants (Knopps, 1993). The children often become part of the delusional thinking, and the woman, in the throes of her psychosis, believes that she and her child have to die. "The disorder is remarkable for its mercurial changeability, and lucid intervals may give a false impression of recovery" (Hamilton, Harberger, & Parry, 1992, p. 35).

PPPs differ from other psychotic episodes because of the change in confusion and cognition. Wisner, Peindl, and Hanusa (1994) compared mothers who had PPP with women with non–childbearing-related psychoses. They reported that compared with the women with non–childbearing-related psychoses, the women with PPPs experienced more symptoms of cognitive impairment and bizarre behavior.

The rate of sleep loss in the triggering of PPP has been alluded to since Hippocrates. Jones (1902) reported that sleep loss was almost a universal early symptom of PPP. Recent studies have found that between 42% and 100% of women with PPP have sleep disturbances (Hunt & Silverstone, 1995; Rohde & Marneros, 1993). Sharma (2003) proposed the role of genetic factors, hormonal changes, and sleep loss in the development of PPP.

Sharma and Mazmanian (2003) warned that a close monitoring of the sleep–wake cycle of mothers who are at high risk of developing PPP is needed. Often sleep loss precedes mania; thus, early identification and treatment of sleep disturbances need to be important parts of managing at risk women such as those with a bipolar disorder or a history of PPP.

Accumulating evidence indicates that a substantial link exists between PPP and bipolar disorder. Jones and Craddock (2001), for example, reported 260 episodes of PPP per 1,000 deliveries in women with bipolar disorders. Chaudron and Pies (2003) urged clinicians to always consider bipolar disorder in their differential diagnosis of any woman presenting with a new onset of affective disorder in the postpartum period, especially if psychotic features are present. Some indications of a possible bipolar diagnosis can include a family history of bipolar disorder or PPP and possible prior mania or hypomania.

In my (Jeanne) clinical experience and that of my colleague Deborah Sichel, we have found that women with PPP may experience psychosis for the first time after the birth of their baby, but there is a positive family history and/or a positive personal history pointing to bipolar sensitivity or susceptibility to mood swing disorders. This again brings home the point that a careful, sensitive history must be obtained before postpartum so that any past disturbances can be identified and considered in the postpartum care plan.

To explore women's experiences of living with PPP, Robertson and Lyons (2003) interviewed 10 mothers who had been diagnosed and treated for PPP. Three major categories were identified: (1) a separate form of mental illness, (2) loss, and (3) relationships and roles. Because childbirth was the cause of the illness, the mothers felt that this set them apart from persons with other forms of mental illness. They perceived that they should be separate and need specialized treatment. Women felt isolated, scared, and like freaks. Adding to their fear was the lack of experience of some clinicians regarding PPP. Women experienced loss in many aspects of their lives, such as loss of control over themselves and decision making regarding their treatment, loss of motherhood and their maternal–child relationships, and loss of enjoying the experience of having more children. PPP placed massive stress on the women's relationships, including those with their spouses. Two higher order concepts of "living with emotions" and "regaining and changing self" emerged across the three main categories. In "living with emotions," the mothers discussed experiencing an array of emotions, particularly feelings of guilt, loss, pain, and fear. In "regaining and changing self," mothers described losing themselves, their minds, and their personalities. Because of their profound and serious mental illness, mothers felt that they were changed. Women believed that PPP had made them stronger. It made them better persons. Their confidence increased, and they felt more sympathetic toward others.

Treatment

PPP is a dangerous illness in that it can lead to infanticide and suicide. It requires aggressive treatment within a hospital setting. The use of mood-stabilizing agents is critical in the treatment plan and needs to be initiated immediately in addition to the antipsychotic medications. Most clinicians recommend the use of the more potent, less sedating, antipsychotic medications such as perphenazine, haloperidol, or fluphenazine. The newer, atypical neuroleptics are holding promise as fast, effective antipsychotic agents (e.g., olanzapine and risperidone). A depression may emerge after the manic/psychosis stage is under control. It is critical that the clinician adds antidepressants in a very gentle, cautious way; if the dose is increased too rapidly, a hypomanic or rapid cycling situation may precipitate.

PPP has about a 90% recurrence rate after the next baby (Kendell et al., 1987). It has been suggested that the administration of prophylaxis with lithium after delivery may prevent recurrence in about 90% of women (Cohen, Sichel, Robertson, Heckscher, & Rosenbaum, 1995; Stewart, Klompenhouwer, Kendell, & van Hulst, 1991).

There is some thought that the rapid drop in estrogen levels implicates a trigger to biochemical brain events that may alter the thyroid and stress hormone levels as well as the dopamine receptors in the brain (Kumar & Robson, 1984). The use of high-dose estrogen in women at risk for early-onset puerperal psychosis may reduce the rate of recurrence; however, high-dose estrogen may increase the risk of thromboembolism at the time when that complication is high otherwise. In light of the fact that mood stabilizers and neuroleptics can be effective in decreasing the risk of recurrence, they are much safer (Cohen et al., 1995; Sichel, Cohen, Roberston, Ruttenberg, & Rosenbaum, 1995).

The prognosis is good for women who experience PPP. In a study conducted by Platz and Kendell (1998), women who experienced PPP were less likely to be readmitted to psychiatric hospitals as compared with women who experienced non-PPP. The postpartum women, if they were hospitalized, spent less time in hospitals compared with the nonpostpartum group.

Case Study

I received a call from a nurse-midwife colleague regarding a patient who she was concerned about. "Jeanne, something is not right. I can't put my finger on it, but she doesn't seem as though she is making sense. She keeps talking about how anxious she is and how afraid she is that they are coming to take her baby away." The woman was 6 days postpartum and was at home with her family. They, too, were concerned and wanted me to see her. An appointment was made for the next day.

Madison was accompanied to my office by her husband, her mother, and her infant, a baby girl, Shannon. Madison looked very frightened and somewhat hesitant to come into my office, although she was holding on to her husband's shirt sleeve. Her mom carried the baby in the infant seat. We got in the room and got seated. I noticed that Madison was looking around with rapid eye movements and looked almost as if she was holding herself together. She turned every so often, as if she was looking or listening to something in the room. Something about her presentation felt a bit psychotic, although I could not describe it. It was more this sense in the back of my head that I have come to trust intuitively. I moved very gently and softly with this assessment, as my primary goal was to establish a connection with Madison so that she could feel a sense of connection and empathy. I started by sharing how I heard from her nurse-midwife, who was a colleague of mine, that she, Madison, seemed to be having a difficult time since the baby was born and that I was a clinical nurse who specialized in the mental health care of new mothers and their babies. Her nurse-midwife thought that it would be a good idea for her to see me. How did she feel about that referral?

Madison looked at me and gently said, "I am so afraid. I don't know what is going on. I feel as though I am going to jump out of my skin, and I just can't settle down." She started to cry. "I am so afraid that they are going to take my baby away from me." I asked her why she thought that, and she said, "because I am a bad mother and I don't deserve this baby." Something was going on inside Madison that was a bit scary—something distant and disconnected, a sense of fear. I could not put my finger on it precisely. In my mind, I really believed that she was psychotic and knew that this consult would probably turn into a focus of hospital admission, but I did my breathing and proceeded forward.

I asked Madison to tell me about her pregnancy with Shannon. She became a bit more focused and smiled and told me, "We had been trying to get pregnant for 3 years. I had all sorts of infertility treatments. Finally, on our second in vitro fertilization, I became pregnant, and here she is." Here were some high-risk indicators in my assessment process: a history of infertility and the use of medications that affected reproductive hormones, stress hormones, and brain neurotransmitters (Figure 4.1). So now what?

"So tell me, Madison, what was it like when you became pregnant? How did you feel then?" I asked. Madison looked deep into my eyes and said, "It was the best time of my life. I was so excited and happy and at the same time anxious and scared that something would happen. Wasn't I, Curt?" (her husband). He looked at her, smiled, and nodded. Madison went on to describe a pregnancy that was full of joy, anxiety, terror, and energy. "After we got past the first trimester and the amnio results were back and I knew she was fine, I was psyched. I love shopping for maternity clothes, baby clothes, and furniture. We painted her room. I was just so excited." The tone of Madison's conversation became higher and more animated as she described the pregnancy. There was a detection of pressure in her speech, and it was a bit rapid. The tone and manner of the communication were other clues that some mania was present. She

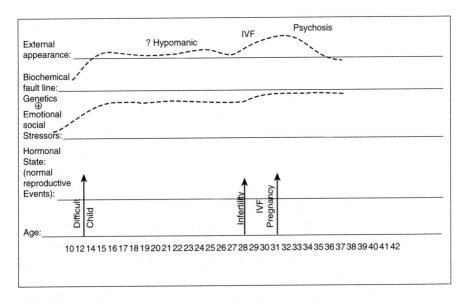

Figure 4.1 The Earthquake Assessment: Madison

Sichel, D. & Driscoll, J.W.: *Women's Moods: What every woman must know about hormones, the brain, and emotional health*. 1999. By permission of HarperCollins Publishers, Inc., p. 100.

described that she continued working as an advertising executive during the pregnancy and worked very hard to have all of her projects in order before she went on maternity leave. Curt began to talk and shared the following: "Madison was flying during the pregnancy. She was so sad while we were trying to get pregnant, a bit depressed I thought, but we kept getting bad news with each cycle. I just figured that that was normal, as I was bummed too. When she finally got pregnant, it was like I had my wife back. She is normally so energetic, focused, and driven and accomplishes so much in a day. I thought she would never come back, but now I am not sure who this person is. She was excited during the pregnancy and even after Shannon was born, but now she just seems so fragile and scared. She seems so distracted all of the time and forgetful. I am really worried about her." Madison's mother picked up the baby out of the infant seat and was patting Shannon and shared, "I am really concerned too." Her eyes were swelling with tears.

Proceeding with the assessment, I asked Shannon to tell me how the birth experience had been for her. Shannon was able to focus and described the labor and delivery process in detail. "I went into labor in my thirty-ninth week. I was ready. I felt so big and uncomfortable. I had contractions beginning on Friday afternoon; they were not too bad, but I called my nurse-midwife. She said to eat lightly, drink fluids, and go on with whatever I was doing and check in with her later to let her know how I was doing. She was on call, which I was glad of because I felt very connected to her. I called her at 11:00 p.m. and told her that the contractions were coming regularly now and that I was feeling a bit anxious and scared. She said that she'd meet us at the hospital. I was so glad to hear that, as I didn't want to be home any longer. Curt and I got to the hospital in about 30 minutes, and Chrissie, my nurse-midwife, was waiting for us. They admitted me to the hospital, started an intravenous, and put the fetal monitor on my belly. Chrissie checked me, and I was 6 centimeters. I was thrilled with that progress, and I didn't think it was as painful as I thought. I was going to go for an unmedicated birth. I had been on so much medication to get pregnant that I really wanted to not take medication if I could avoid it to give birth." She went on to describe the labor as she moved through transition and the second stage with pushing. "I felt so empowered and so excited that I could be that connected to the process of pushing out my much wanted baby." The baby was born after 1.5 hours of pushing. "She was beautiful; I just laughed and cried when I saw her. They put her right on my belly. Curt cut the cord. She was looking right at me. I was in love, and she was wonderful." Curt talked about how excited they both were and how they called their parents to tell them of Shannon's arrival while they were still in the labor room. "We were all so excited. We had waited so long for this baby girl to come into our lives," said Curt, as he looked at the baby in his mother-in-law's arms.

The first day after Shannon was born was fantastic. "I was flying. I was so happy. I had so much energy. I had no medication, a small episiotomy. I had my baby. The nurses were telling me to rest and take a nap. I couldn't. I was just so excited and energized. Shannon took to the breast right away, and I was in awe. I would sit and stare at her. Curt stayed with me in the hospital. All of the family came that day and brought champagne and baby gifts. What a celebration!" They went home the next day. "I just started to feel tired and strange. Something broke inside me, and I don't know what it is." Madison become quiet now and looked a bit preoccupied by something else. I gently asked her, "Madison, where are you?" My question caused her to refocus at me. She looked at me and said, "Did you hear that?" I asked her what she heard. "That voice—someone is telling me to get out of here. Did you hear it?" I replied that I had not heard that and asked whether she had heard this voice before. "Yes, it keeps coming and going. I keep trying to push it away. It is as if it follows me around. I have this thought that I have to get rid of the baby or something bad is going to happen to me and her." At this point, her husband and her mother looked panicked. Their eyes were a wide as saucers, and they looked at me quickly. I asked Madison whether this voice had told her to harm her baby. "It keeps telling me that she has to go away or something bad is going to happen. I just give the baby to my mother or Curt. I don't want to do anything to her. What is going on? Where is this voice coming from?" I asked Madison how long she had been hearing the voice. It started the day they come home from the hospital, and she just kept trying to keep busy or to sleep, "although I can't sleep at all."

I asked Madison if she had ever heard this voice before in her life or if she ever had times when she felt too energetic, wound up, rageful, agitated, drank too much, spent too much money, or anything impulsive or out of character. Madison was able to answer the questions in between periods of looking disconnected and like she had left the room mentally. I figured that it was at those times that she was hearing that voice again. I asked Curt and her mother to help me with some more history, as I saw that it was getting harder on Madison.

Madison's mother shared with me that she had a son, Madison's brother, who had been diagnosed with bipolar disorder a few years ago and that he was doing well on lithium. Her husband had never been diagnosed with a mood disorder, but she believes that he, too, has a sort of manic-depressive illness, as he gets very involved in projects and then just tuckers out and does not finish them. When the children were young, he was easily irritated and angered. She used to pray that he would not come home until they were in bed. She wanted to protect them from him and his agitated behavior. He drank two manhattans every night, and she felt that kept him calm in the evening. Madison's sister was in therapy, and there was some talk that she had a mood disorder, too. However, she was not on any medications at this time.

When Madison was growing up, she was a difficult child. "She was very intense and moody. She would flip at the switch of the light—unpredictable. When she was good, she was very good, but when she would have those episodes of in-your-face hostility, living with her was very hard." Madison, as described by her mother, was very intelligent and was in the gifted and talented program. She excelled in high school and studied very hard, often late into the night. She graduated with honors, and in college, she was Phi Beta Kappa. Madison was very goal directed and intense and achieved whatever goals she had.

Curt described that Madison's intense and goal-oriented personality was what had drawn him to her. She was exciting, energetic, focused, and successful and a lot of fun. He put his arm around her and looked at her and said, "I feel in love with this ball of energy, and I love her intensely. Now I am very worried because this isn't her. Is it Madison? Something is wrong, and you have to help us."

I looked at them all while observing Madison. "Madison, I believe that you are experiencing a PPP. This is treatable and recoverable. You are going to be okay. We just have to take care of you and your brain." I described that PPP was a form of bipolar illness that occurred after the birth of a baby and that it occurs in 1 to 2 cases per 1,000 women who give birth. Madison's family history of bipolar illnesses, her response to infertility medications, and the estrogen of the pregnancy were high-risk signs that she probably was living with a mood-swing disorder but had been able to cope and adjust her life accordingly. However, with the rapid drop of the estrogen/progesterone hormones in the postpartum period, her brain biochemistry dysregulated, leading to the symptoms that she was now experiencing. I really felt that Madison would benefit from being admitted to the psychiatric unit so that she could receive medication and be able to focus on self-care. She would not be in hospital very long. Her mother and husband looked at me with what felt like a mix of terror and relief.

While they were in my office, I called their insurance company to find out what hospital systems were in their network and made a call to the psychiatric admission office. Fortunately, a bed was available in the necessary unit. Madison was crying and shaking in Curt's arms. Her mother was just rocking the baby, and tears were falling down her cheeks. I shared with them again that this was treatable and that she would be fine. We just had to get her on some medications to re-regulate her brain biochemistry. The initial medications were a class called the atypical neuroleptics: Risperdal (risperidone), Zyprexa (olanzapine), and Seroquel (quetiapine). These medications would help take away the voices that she was hearing. She would be started on mood stabilizers, most likely lithium, as that had worked for her brother. We talked about the breastfeeding. We would arrange to get a breast pump for use while in the hospital. Our goal was not to take that away but to preserve that process. We would discuss breastfeeding after her symptoms were under control. There are some ongoing studies of lithium use and breast milk, and after she could make some decisions, we would discuss that (Altshuler, et al, 2002).

The four of them left my office, and she was admitted that night. After about 4 days in the hospital, Madison was discharged and continued her care with me in the private practice setting. She did very well on lithium and a low-dose neuroleptic at bedtime. She chose not to continue breastfeeding but weaned in a physiologic manner with the breast pump and good support. Her therapy focused in the early weeks on why this happened and how to deal with feelings of guilt, grief, loss, and anger at the entire process. Today, Madison, Curt, and Shannon are doing well. They are hoping to have another baby. We will work closely together to support and promote a healthy pregnancy and postpartum experience.

References

Altshuler, L.L., Cohen, L.S., Moline, M.L., Kahn, D.A., Carpenter, D., Docherty, J.P., & Ross, R.W. (2002). Expert consensus guidelines for the treatment of depression in women: A new treatment tool. MentalFitness, 1, 69–83.

American Psychological Association. (2004). Diagnostic and statistical manual of mental disorders (4th Ed.) Text revision. Washington, DC: Author.

Appleby, L., & Mortensen, P. B., & Faragher, E. B. (1998). Suicide and other causes of mortality after post-partum psychiatric admission. British Journal of Psychiatry, 173, 209–211.

Brockington, I. F., Cernick, K. F., Schofield, E. M., Downing, A. R., Francis, A. F., & Keelan, C. (1981). Puerperal psychosis. *Archives in General Psychiatry, 38*, 829–833.

Chaudron, L. H., & Pies, R. W. (2003). The relationship between postpartum psychosis and bipolar disorders: A review. *Journal of Clinical Psychiatry, 64*, 1284–1292.

Cohen, L. S., Sichel, D. A., Robertson, L. M., Heckscher, E., & Rosenbaum, J. F. (1995). Postpartum prophylaxis for women with bipolar disorder. *The American Journal of Psychiatry, 152*(11), 1641–1645.

Hamilton, J. A., Harberger, P. N., & Parry B. L. (1992). The problem of terminology. In J. A. Hamilton & P. N. Harberger (Eds.), *Postpartum psychiatric illness: A picture puzzle* (pp. 33–40). Philadelphia: University of Pennsylvania Press.

Hunt, N., & Silverstone, T. (1995). Does puerperal illness distinguish a subgroup of bipolar parents? *Journal of Affective Disorders, 34*, 101–107.

Jones, R. (1902). Puerperal insanity. *British Medical Journal, 1*, 576–585.

Jones, I., & Craddock, N. (2001). Familiarity of the puerperal trigger in bipolar disorder: Results of a family study. *American Journal of Psychiatry, 158*, 913–917.

Kendell, R., Chalmers, J., & Platz, C. (1987). Epidemiology of puerperal psychosis. *British Journal of Psychiatry, 150*, 662–673.

Knopps, G. G. (1993). Postpartum mood disorders: A startling contrast to the joy of birth. *Postgraduate Medicine, 93*, 103–116.

Kumar, R. C., & Robson, K. (1984). A prospective study of emotional disorders in childbearing women. *British Journal of Psychiatry, 144*, 37–45.

McGorry, P., & Connell, S. (1990). The nosology and prognosis of puerperal psychosis: A review. *Comprehensive Psychiatry, 31*, 519–534.

Platz, C., & Kendell, R. E. (1988). A matched-control follow-up and family study of "puerperal" psychosis. *British Journal of Psychiatry, 114*, 90–94.

Robertson, E., & Lyons, A. (2003). Living with puerperal psychosis: A qualitative analysis. *Psychology and Psychotherapy: Theory, Research, and Practice, 76*, 411–431.

Rohde, A., & Marneros, A. (1993). Postpartum psychoses: Onset and long-term course. *Psychopathology, 26*, 203–209.

Sharma, V. (2003). Role of sleep loss in the causation of puerperal psychosis. *Medical Hypotheses, 61*, 477–481.

Sharma, V., & Mazmanian, D. (2003). Sleep loss and postpartum psychosis. *Bipolar Disorders, 5*, 98–105.

Sichel, D. A., Cohen, L. S., Roberston, L. M., Ruttenberg, A., & Rosenbaum, J. F. (1995). Prophylactic estrogen in recurrent postpartum affective disorder. *Biological Psychiatry, 38*, 814–818.

Stewart, D. E., Klompenhouwer, J. L., Kendell, R. E., & van Hulst, A. M. (1991). Prophylactic lithium in puerperal psychosis—the experience of three centers. *British Journal of Psychiatry, 158*, 393–397.

Wisner, K. L., Peindl, K. S., & Hanusa, B. H. (1994). Symptomatology and affective and psychotic illness related to childbearing. *Journal of Affective Disorders, 20*, 77–87.

CHAPTER 5

POSTPARTUM DEPRESSION

Criteria for Major Depressive Episode

A. Five (or more) of the following symptoms have been present during the same 2-week period and represent a change from previous functioning; at least one of the symptoms is either (1) depressed mood or (2) a loss of interest or pleasure.

Note: Do not include symptoms that are clearly caused by a general medical condition or mood-incongruent delusions or hallucinations.

1. Depressed mood most of the day, nearly every day, as indicated by either subjective report (e.g., feels sad or empty) or observation made by others (e.g., appears tearful)

2. Markedly diminished interest or pleasure in all, or almost all, activities most of the day, nearly every day (as indicated by either subjective account or observation made by others)

3. Significant weight loss when not dieting or weight gain (e.g., a change of more than 5% of body weight in a month) or a decrease or increase in appetite nearly every day

4. Insomnia or hypersomnia nearly every day

5. Psychomotor agitation or retardation nearly every day (observable by others, not merely subjective feelings of restlessness or being slowed down)

6. Fatigue or loss of energy nearly every day

7. Feelings of worthlessness or excessive or inappropriate guilt (which may be delusional) nearly every day (not merely self-reproach or guilt about being sick)

8. A diminished ability to think or concentrate or indecisiveness nearly every day (either by subjective account or as observed by others)
9. Recurrent thoughts of death (not just fear of dying), recurrent suicidal ideation without a specific plan, or a suicide attempt or a specific plan for committing suicide
B. The symptoms do not meet criteria for a mixed episode.
C. The symptoms cause clinically significant distress or impairment in social, occupational, or other important areas of functioning.
D. The symptoms are not due to the direct physiologic effects of a substance (e.g., a drug of abuse, a medication) or a general medical condition (e.g., hypothyroidism).
E. The symptoms are not better accounted for by bereavement; that is, after the loss of a loved one, the symptoms persist for longer than 2 months or are characterized by marked functional impairment, morbid preoccupation with worthlessness, suicidal ideation, psychotic symptoms, or psychomotor retardation. (American Psychiatric Association, 2000, p. 356)

Criteria for Postpartum Onset Specifier

Specify if:

With postpartum onset (can be applied to the current or most recent major depressive, manic, or mixed episode in major depressive disorder, bipolar I disorder, or bipolar II disorder; or to brief psychotic disorder), onset of episode within 4 weeks postpartum (American Psychiatric Association, 2000, p. 423).

Reprinted with permission from the *Diagnostic and Statistical Manual of Mental Disorders*, Copyright 2000. American Psychiatric Association.

Introduction

This chapter focuses on postpartum depression. Because a large amount of material is covered, the chapter is divided into sections. First, the risk factors for postpartum depression are identified, followed by the epidemiology of this mood disorder. Cultural influences and the phenomenology of postpartum depression are then covered. Next, postpartum depression in adoptive mothers, pregnancy loss, and fathers is described.

Attention is then focused on the effects of this crippling mood disorder on mothers' interactions with their infants and also on their children's cognitive and emotional development. Toward the end of the chapter, treatment takes center stage, and secondary interventions and psychopharmacologic treatments are presented. The chapter ends with a case study and its related NURSE program.

Postpartum depression affects 10% to 15% of women after the birth of their baby (O'Hara & Swain, 1996). Clinically, the rates are higher, because a major issue with the data collection of occurrence of the diagnosis has to do with the labeling and the operational definition of "postpartum." As discussed earlier, the American Psychiatric Association (2000) defines the term postpartum as 4 weeks after the birth of a baby. Sadly, this onset descriptor is often too limiting for the time experience of the onset of this disorder. Postpartum depression, although not found to be a distinct diagnosis, is indeed unique in the context of its occurrence. The woman is experiencing symptoms of a major depressive disorder during the developmental life event of birthing and/or adopting a child. She is in the middle of an experience in which she is responsible for the care of a dependent human being who cannot feed himself/herself or roll over without assistance. She is forced to focus her care and attention to this dependent baby, and at the same time, she is struggling with symptoms of depression that are getting in the way of her everyday living. Sadly, the context experience of postpartum in the United States culture is laden with preconceived notions, performance expectations, and Madison Avenue–marketed images. This is not the reality.

As discussed in the maternity blues chapter, the reality of normal postpartum adjustment is an experience that is laden with insecurities, fears, concerns, and a myriad of emotions. The experience of living with the baby and the process of becoming a mother is rarely discussed or marketed in the media. It is the underground network of women where the initiation is that you have a child. Once you are in the club, as they say, the truth comes out, and women tend to share their truths. We live in a culture in which you are encouraged to look good and speak only good, nice things. The reality is that having a baby and becoming a mother is a life-changing event: psychologically, physically, culturally, spiritually, and emotionally. A woman's world changes. As the woman becomes a member of the secret society, there are covert agreements and knowing nods. Society does not want to hear the reality of the experience, which is that the experience of having a baby and learning to become a mother are a total experience and a life-altering event. It can be a time of significant growth and self-awareness. It is a time when many women are able to reassess and become self-aware, self-confident, and authentic.

Experiencing postpartum depression can be a "gift" as part of the recovery process in that the woman takes time to care for herself. The recovery from the illness makes this self-focused approach critical. She learns that if she does not take care of herself, then not many emotional reserves are left over to support, care, and raise her child. Very often when sitting with new mothers in the midst of postpartum depression and we tell them that this experience will ultimately be a gift to them, they look at us like we are crazy. However, about a year later when we meet again, they often will say, "When you said this would be a gift, now I really understand what you meant."

Postpartum Depression Risk Factors

Identifying a woman's risk factors or predictors of postpartum depression is critical. Obviously, the best intervention for this devastating mood disorder is to prevent it from happening in the first place. Interventions can be initiated before the onset of postpartum depression in hopes of preventing its occurrence. The period before delivery is a perfect time to begin: the earlier the better. Even if a woman has already developed postpartum depression, it is not too late to identify her risk factors. Dealing with individual risk factors can become part of the treatment plan for her postpartum depression.

In order to summarize quantitatively the results of research conducted on predictors of postpartum depression, meta-analyses have been conducted (Beck, 1996, 2001; O'Hara & Swain, 1996). O'Hara and Swain determined the strength of the magnitude of risk factors for postpartum depression that had been measured during pregnancy. Effect sizes were reported as Cohen's (1988) d indicators, with a d of 0.2 indicating a small relationship, 0.4 indicating a medium relationship, and 0.8 or more indicating a strong relationship. The strongest predictors of postpartum depression in O'Hara and Swain's meta-analysis were prenatal depression ($d = 0.75$), prenatal anxiety ($d = 0.68$), social support ($d = -0.63$), life events ($d = 0.60$), and the mother's history of psychopathology ($d = 0.57$). The meta-analysis revealed the following three predictors that had small, significant relationships with postpartum depression: neuroticism ($d = 0.39$), negative cognitive attributional style ($d = 0.24$), and obstetric variables ($d = 0.26$).

I conducted a meta-analysis to determine the magnitude of the relationships between various predictor variables and postpartum depression (Beck, 1996a). Effect sizes were reported as Cohen's r indicators, with r = 0.10 being small, r = 0.30 being medium, and r = 0.50 or more being large. The strongest predictor of this mood disorder was prenatal depression, which had a large effect size (r = 0.51). Moderate effect sizes were revealed for the relationships between postpartum depression and the following predictors: childcare stress (r = 0.48), life stress (r = 0.40), low social support (r = 0.38), prenatal anxiety (r = 0.35), maternity blues (r = 0.36), and marital dissatisfaction (r = 0.35). Finally, a history of previous depression was shown to have a small effect size (r = 0.29) when determining its relationship with postpartum depression. In a different meta-analysis (Beck, 1996b), infant temperament was also revealed to be a significant predictor of postpartum depression.

Since these meta-analyses had been published, the number of studies investigating predictors of postpartum depression had greatly increased; thus, in 2001, the 1996a meta-analysis was replicated by Cheryl and included studies published throughout the 1990s (Beck, 2001). This updated meta-analysis revealed 13 significant predictors of postpartum depression (Table 5.1). Of the 13 significant predictors for postpartum depression, 10 of these risk factors had moderate effect sizes: prenatal depression, low self-esteem, childcare stress, prenatal anxiety, life stress, low social support, poor marital relationship, history of depression, infant temperament, and maternity blues. Three predictors had small effect sizes:

Table 5.1   THIRTEEN SIGNIFICANT PREDICTORS OF POSTPARTUM DEPRESSION FROM BECK'S 2001 META-ANALYSIS

Predictor	Interpretation of Effect Size
Prenatal depression	Medium
Child care stress	Medium
Life stress	Medium
Social support	Medium
Prenatal anxiety	Medium
Marital dissatisfaction	Medium
Depression history	Medium
Infant temperament	Medium
Maternity blues	Small/medium
Self-esteem	Medium
Socioeconomic status	Small
Marital status	Small
Unplanned/unwanted pregnancy	Small

marital status, socioeconomic (SES), and unplanned/unwanted pregnancy. The strongest postpartum depression risk factors were prenatal depression, low self-esteem, childcare stress, and prenatal anxiety. The effect sizes of these four risk factors closely approached Cohen's (1988) cutoff for a large effect size. The three risk factors of maternity blues, childcare stress, and infant temperament were specific to only the postpartum period, whereas the other 10 predictors were also operant during pregnancy.

All 13 significant predictors of postpartum depression identified through Beck's (2001) meta-analysis fit under the umbrella of Sichel and Driscoll's (1999) earthquake model. These risk factors can repeatedly weaken a mother's fault line, placing her in a dangerous position for an emotional earthquake. The replicated meta-analysis (Beck, 2001) also confirmed some findings from O'Hara and Swain's (1996) meta-analysis. They reported that the strongest risk factors of postpartum depression were a past history of psychopathology, psychiatric disturbance during pregnancy, a poor marital relationship, low social support, and stressful life events. Low socioeconomic status was found to have a small but significant predictive relationship. Three risk factors that displayed significant relationships with postpartum depression in the replicated meta-analysis that were not found in O'Hara and Swain's meta-analytic review were low self-esteem, single marital status, and unplanned/unwanted pregnancy.

Two of these new risk factors of postpartum depression are demographic variables: marital status and socioeconomic status. These predictors help to sketch out a beginning demographic profile of vulnerable mothers who tend to be unmarried and have low household incomes. These women at risk for this postpartum mood disorder may experience multiple stressors, such as financial difficulties, related to their demographic status that is exacerbated after delivery. Single, low-income women may have fewer resources to help manage the transition to parenthood.

Based on research in the 1990s, low self-esteem has emerged not only as a new, significant predictor of this postpartum mood disorder but also as one of the strongest. Self-esteem may help to buffer the negative effects of stressful life events (Orozco, 1995). Women with high self-esteem may be able to withstand stressors that can jeopardize this sense of self-worth and contribute to the development of postpartum depression. Heath care providers, however, should not be lulled into a false sense of security if a woman does possess a high level of self-esteem. In their model of women's mental health, Sichel and Driscoll (1999) warned that the postpartum period "is a fragile time for the self-esteem of the ablest women and is made much worse by the occurrence of a depression" (p. 198).

Researchers in Canada conducted the most recent meta-analysis on prenatal risk factors for postpartum depression (Robertson, Grace, Wallington, & Stewart, 2004). The strongest predictors of this mood disorder included prenatal depression, prenatal anxiety, stressful life events, low levels of social support, and a previous history of depression. Moderate predictors were poor marital relationship and neuroticism. Obstetric factors and low socioeconomic factors were small predictors.

Significant risk factors of postpartum depression can be used by clinicians as markers or red flags that a mother may be at risk for developing this crippling mood disorder. Specific interventions can then be designed to fit the profile of risk factors for each specific mother. Consistent evidence is accumulating that these same predictors are significant around the globe. For example, in Finland, postpartum depression was predicted by prenatal depression and prenatal anxiety (Saisto, Salmela-Aro, Nurmi, & Halmesmaki, 2001). In Australia, stressful life events, a past history of depression, a poor marital relationship, and low social support were significantly related to postpartum depression (Boyce, 2003).

Evidence is mounting that mothers of preterm infants and those who experience multiple births experience a higher rate of postpartum depression than women who deliver full-term singleton infants. Depression and anxiety disorders are more prevalent in mothers of multiples, affecting over 25% of these mothers during the prenatal and postpartum periods (Leonard, 1998). The high incidence of preterm deliveries, sleep deprivation, social isolation, and the constant demands of the twins may contribute to depression in families of multiples. One research team followed mothers of twins 5 years after delivery and reported that 34% of mothers who had two living twins and 53% of women who had only one living twin were clinically depressed (Thorpe, Golding, MacGillivray, & Greenwood, 1991). Cheryl's grounded theory study of mothering twins over the first year of life revealed that the most vulnerable time for the onset of postpartum depression was the first 3 months after delivery, with 19% of the mothers experiencing postpartum depression compared with the usual rate of 13% (Beck, 2002).

The stress associated with multiple births frequently is compounded by a premature delivery. This is significant because mothers of preterm infants experience a higher level of depression than mothers of full-term infants (Logsdon, Davis, Birkimer, & Wilkerson, 1997; Veddovi, Kerry, Gibson, Bowen, & Starte, 2001). Mothers of preterm infants (n = 37), who were assessed for postpartum depression shortly before their infants' neonatal intensive care unit (NICU) discharge and again at their infant's 4-week follow-up visit, were frequently depressed at this 1-month visit

(Logsdon et al., 1997). Low social support and low self-esteem were predictive. High levels of depression at 1- and 12-months postpartum were reported in a longitudinal study of 69 Hispanic mothers of very low birth weight infants. Social support appeared to buffer the effects of depression in the sample.

Davis, Edwards, Mohay, and Wollin (2003) investigated the impact of very premature birth on the psychologic health of mothers. Using the Edinburgh Postnatal Depression Scale (EPDS) (Cox, Holden, & Sagovsky, 1987), Davis et al. reported that 40% of 62 mothers of very preterm infants had significant depressive symptoms. Also using the EPDS, Drewett, Blair, Emmett, Emond, and the Avon Longitudinal Study of Parents and Children (ALSPAC) study team (2004) reported that preterm births were specifically associated with higher maternal depression scores in the postpartum period than mothers of full-term infants.

Known postpartum depression predictors, such as child care stress, have been examined in parents of NICU infants. In a descriptive study (n = 212 parents of NICU infants), the mothers' perceptions of the severity of their infant's illness was the strongest factor related to their parental stress scores (Shields-Poe & Pinelli, 1997). Low social support, another known predictor of postpartum depression, was documented in a study of 37 mothers of hospitalized preterm infants that examined the types of support mothers expected and received after their infants' discharge from the NICU (Davis, Logsdon, & Birkmer, 1996). These mothers reported less material, emotional, and informational support than they had expected. Depressive symptoms at the time of NICU discharge were evaluated in 30 mothers of preterm infants (Veddovi et al., 2001). Maternal depressive symptoms were predicted by less accurate knowledge of infant development. These researchers suggest that educating mothers of preterm infants about infant development may provide protection against the development of postpartum depression.

Epidemiology of Postpartum Depression

Hendrick, Altshulter, Strouse, and Grosser (2000) reported that the onset of postpartum depression usually occurs within the first 4 weeks after birth. Small, Brown, Lumley, and Astbury (1994) reported that almost 50% of depressed mothers began their depression within the first 3 months postpartum, whereas a third more developed depression after 3 months postpartum.

Goodman (2004) reviewed the literature for the 20-year period of 1982 to 2002. Studies were included that measured postpartum depression or postpartum depressive symptomatology at one or more times from 6 months to 2.5 years after childbirth. She concluded that postpartum depression and depressive symptoms remain problematic for a significant number of mothers into the second half of the first 12 months after delivery. Goodman identified that in community samples the point prevalence of postpartum depression at 6 months after birth ranged from 9.1% to 38.2%.

In the Agency for Healthcare Research and Quality's (AHRQ) evidence report (Gaynes et al., 2005) point prevalence of major depression alone was highest at 2 months postpartum (5.7%) and 6 months postpartum (5.6%). For major and minor depression the point prevalence was highest at 3 months postpartum (12.9%), then it decreased slightly in the fourth through seventh month after delivery (9.9–10.6%).

Current research from a variety of countries revealed that a significant percentage of mothers are depressed at 6 months after giving birth. In the United States, 35% of mothers were depressed (Beeghly et al., 2002) at this time, whereas 54% of the sample in Zelkowitz and Milet's (2001) sample at 6 months postpartum were still depressed in Canada. At 6 months after birth, 13% of the mothers in a Swedish study remained depressed (Josefsson, Berg, Nordin, & Sydsjo, 2001).

At 6 to 12 months postpartum, 15% of an Australian sample of mothers scored 13 or above on the EPDS (Cox et al., 1987; Hiscock & Wake, 2001). In the United States, 24% of the sample at 12 months after delivery were still diagnosed with having major postpartum depression (Campbell & Cohn, 1977). The period prevalence of elevated postpartum depressive symptoms during the first 12 months after childbirth has ranged from 24% (Kumar & Robson, 1984) to 27.3% (Matthey, Barnett, Ungerer, & Waters, 2000).

Kendell, Chalmers, and Platz's (1987) classic large epidemiologic study showed an increase in the rate of psychiatric admissions in the first 3 months postpartum, with a definite peak in the first months after delivery. Of the 257 mothers who had psychiatric admissions to hospitals in the first 12 months after childbirth, 68 (26%) were admitted during the first 30 days postpartum.

The timing and pattern of recurrence of depression during the first year after birth in women with a history of prior episodes of postpartum major depression were studied prospectively (Wisner, Perel, Peindl, & Hanusa, 2004). Fifty-one women who had at least one past episode of postpartum depression were recruited during their pregnancies to participate in the study. After delivery, mothers were evaluated every week for 20 weeks and then at 24-, 36-, and 52-weeks postpartum with the Hamilton Rating Scale for Depression and the Research Diagnostic Criteria. Of the 51 women, 21 had recurrences of major postpartum depression (41%). Nineteen of the 21 recurrences occurred in the first 28 weeks postpartum. The remaining two cases occurred at weeks 50 and 52.

Culture

In the 1980s, the debate began over whether postpartum depression was a Western culture-bound syndrome. Stern and Kruckman (1983, p. 1036) hypothesized "that the negative outcomes of depression and baby blues in the U.S. result from the relative lack of (1) social structuring of postpartum events; (2) social recognition of a role transition for the new mother; and (3) instrumental assistance to the new mother."

Stern and Kruckman identified six necessary components of postpartum activities, which provide social support for new mothers and help to buffer or prevent postpartum depression. These basic components were as follows (1983, p. 1039):

1. Structuring of a distinct postpartum time period
2. Protective measures and rituals reflecting the presumed vulnerability of the new mother
3. Social seclusion
4. Mandated rest
5. Assistance in tasks from relatives and/or midwife
6. Social recognition through rituals, gifts, etc., after new social status of the mother.

Seel (1986) also argued that rituals and customs surrounding birth and the postpartum period are critical for a mother to feel that her new role is valued by her culture and that a supporting network of family and friends surround her. Bhugra and Gregorie (1993) proposed four basic themes within these protective rituals: (1) isolating and secluding the new mother, (2) intensive caring and support of the new mother, (3) behavioral proscriptions on the women such as "doing the month" among the Chinese (Pillsbury, 1978) or dietary restrictions, and (4) suspending of social roles and protecting from previous demands.

In "doing the month," Chinese mothers receive extra attention and help from their families during the month after delivery. Pillsbury (1978) described how during these 30 days Chinese mothers follow set rules of behavior, such as not going outside, not eating any raw or cold food, and avoiding washing. Pillsbury concluded that this extra attention and rest might prevent Chinese women from having postpartum depression. Seel (1986) regarded these childbirth rituals as "rites de passage" and when incomplete, as in Western society, relate to an increase in postpartum depression. Seel purported that in the Western society the mother and father are left in limbo. New parents are left to fend for themselves as best they can. Without these rituals, mothers are stripped of protective layers. This cultural stereotyping is dangerous, however, because of the possibility that postpartum depression in non-Western culture may go unrecognized (Kumar, 1994).

Cox (1979, 1983) in his ground-breaking research with new mothers from the Ganda tribe in Southern Uganda revealed that postpartum depression did exist in non-Western cultures and at similar rates as those in developed countries. Cox (1979) described *Amakiro*, which is a serious mental illness after childbirth. It at times resulted in the death of the mother or her infant. Mothers suffering from *Amakiro* displayed a disordered relationship with the infants. Mothers, for instance, did not want to feed their babies. In another pioneering transcultural study, Cox (1983) compared the rates of postpartum depression in two samples: one in Scotland and one in Uganda. The frequency of this postpartum mood disorder was remarkably similar. In Uganda, Cox reported that 10% of the mothers had postpartum depression compared with 13% of the mothers in Scotland. The only minor difference between mothers between these two cultures was that the Scottish women were more likely to report that they felt personally responsible for the infants and that they felt guilty or self-blame.

Now, after 20 years of transcultural research on postpartum depression, evidence is accumulating that the prevalence of this postpartum mood disorder is fairly consistent globally. In Cox's (1983) study, for example, semirural African women with postpartum depression were readily identified, illustrating that this disorder is not confined to Western cultures and is not the result of stripping away of the traditional rituals of new motherhood in developed Western cultures. Table 5.2 includes rates of diagnosed postpartum depression, and Table 5.3 includes rates of elevated postpartum depressive symptomatology.

Oates et al. (2004) explored whether postpartum depression is a universal experience with common attributions and how it is described. The research occurred in 11 countries: France, Ireland, Italy, Sweden, United States, Uganda, United Kingdom, Japan, Portugal, Austria, and Switzerland. Three different groups participated in this qualitative study: new mothers, relatives, and health care professionals. "Morbid unhappiness" (postpartum depression) was recognized by participants in all 11 countries as a common experience after delivery. In most countries, the term "postnatal depression" was used to describe this phenomenon. This term was not used, however, in Portugal, Switzerland, or Uganda or by the UK Asians. The characteristics of postpartum depression were described, however, in all of the countries and were closely related to the Western concept of nonpsychotic depression. In most countries, low social support, family conflict, a lack of sleep, and problems with the baby were identified as causes of postnatal depression.

Qualitative research is needed to examine the profile of postpartum depressive symptoms in mothers across cultures. One such study investigated the

Table 5.2   INTERNATIONAL RATES OF POSTPARTUM DEPRESSION

AUTHORS	COUNTRY	PREVALENCE (%)	PPD
Nhiwatiwa, Patel, and Acuda (1998)	Zimbabwe	16	RCIS Standard psychiatric interview
Regmi, Sligl, Carter, Grut, and Seear (2002)	Katmandu (Nepal)	12	DSM-IV
Chandran, Thoryan, Muliyil, and Abraham (2002)	Tamil Nadu, India	11	CIS-R
Lee, Yip, Chiu, Leung, and Chung (2001)	Hong Kong	12	DSM-IV
Yamashita, Yoshida, Nakano, and Tashiro (2000)	Kyushu, Japan	17	SADS
Rahman, Iqbal, and Harrington (2003)	Pakistan	28	SCAN
Wolf, DeAndraca, and Lozoff (2002)	Costa Rica (2 samples)	40–48	DIS
Patel, Rodrigues, and Desouza (2002)	Goa, India	23	RCIS
Carpiniello, Pariante, Serri, Costa, and Carta (1997)	Italy	15	PSE
Beck and Gable (2005)	Hispanics in the United States	37	DSM-IV

experiences of 35 Hong Kong Chinese women diagnosed with postpartum depression. Chan, Levy, Chung, and Lee (2002) conducted a qualitative study. Four themes emerged from these interviews. These themes were (1) trapped in the situation, (2) ambivalent toward the baby, (3) uncaring husband, and (4) controlling and powerful in-laws. The central theme focused on mothers' feelings of entrapment. Women diagnosed with postpartum depression were anxious, angry, confused, and tired. Mothers suffered with a loss of control over their emotions and behavior. Guilt over their feelings toward their babies and their ability to take care of the infants consumed mothers. All of these themes that were shared by Chinese mothers are the same as those that mothers in the United States experienced (Beck, 1993). The only difference was the last theme

Table 5.3 INTERNATIONAL RATES OF POSTPARTUM DEPRESSIVE SYMPTOMS

Authors	Country	Prevalence (%)	Symptoms
Inandi et al. (2002)	Turkey	27.2	EPDS
Bugdayci, Sasmaz, Tezcan, Kurt, and Oner (2004)	Turkey	29–36.6	EPDS
Felice, Saliba, Grech, and Cox (2004)	Malta	8.7	EPDS
Huang and Mathers (2001)	United Kingdom	18	
	Taiwan	19	EPDS
Danaci, Dinc, Deveci, Sen, and Icelli (2002)	Turkey	14	EPDS
Chaaya et al. (2002)	Beirut, Lebanon	21	EPDS
Affonso, De, Horowitz, and Mayberry (2000)	Sweden	15.2	
	Australia	16	
	Finland	20.7	
	Italy	24	
	USA	29.5	
	India	32.4	
	Korea	36.1	
	Guyana	57	
	Taiwan	60.8	
	All	33.6	EPDS

of controlling and powerful in-laws. The American women did not address this theme at all as a component of their postpartum depression experience.

Amankwaa (2003) described the nature of postpartum depression among 12 African American women. The basic process that mothers used to cope with their devastating mood disorder was entitled "enduring." For these mothers, enduring referred to their holding up under the pain, fatigue, and distress to survive their depression after the birth of their infants. Six themes represented aspects of African American mothers' experiences of postpartum depression: "stressing out," "feeling down," "losing it," "seeking help," "feeling better," and "dealing with it." This last theme of "dealing with it" focused on the cultural ways that these women coped with their postpartum depression: keeping the faith, trying to be a strong black woman, living with myths, and keeping secrets.

An illness narrative was conducted with 19 mothers in Goa, India, who were suffering from postpartum depression (Rodrigues, Patel, Jaswal, & de Souza, 2003) to examine the cultural validity of the concept of postpartum depression in non-Western societies. The symptoms experienced by the postpartum depressed Indian mothers were similar to those found in research with mothers in other cultures. Rodrigues et al. suggested that this is evidence supporting a universal clinical presentation of postpartum depression. The Indian mothers shared that a lack of practical support was a factor contributing to this mood disorder after delivery. Postpartum depressed women expressed the need for more emotional support. These women shared that they had strained relationships with their husbands and in-laws because of the infant's gender. Symptoms reported by the Indian women suffering from postpartum depression included headaches, sleeping problems, worries, crying, giddy/dizziness, self-harm thoughts, tension, nervousness, no interest in doing anything, fatigue, loss of appetite, irritable, angry, sad, feeling strange, and body aches. Mothers interpreted this postpartum depression not from a biomedical psychiatric model but from the context of poor marital relationships and economic difficulties.

The relationship between depressive symptoms and social support in Taiwanese women "doing the month" after childbirth was explored by Heh, Coombes, and Bartlett (2004). The sample consisted of 178 mothers who completed the EPDS and the Postpartum Social Support Questionnaire during the fourth week after giving birth. The higher the level of dissatisfaction with parents' instrumental support received by Taiwanese mothers during the month after birth, the higher the level of depressive symptoms. Twenty-one percent of the sample had EPDS scores indicative of high levels of depressive symptomatology. Heh et al. (2004) concluded that their findings support the thesis that the prevalence of postpartum depression does not appear to vary across different cultures.

White (2004) conducted an ethnographic study in Cambodia to discover the postpartum beliefs and practices of Khmer women. Findings came from 11 focus group discussions with 88 Khmer women of child-bearing age and interviews with 21 Khmer women and 20 birth attendants. The concept of *toas* refers to postpartum complications. One type of *toas* comes from strong emotions and is called *pruey cet*, which means "sad heart." The major symptom of this *toas* was depression or unhappiness. Most of the women in the study believed that *pruey cet* was caused by "thinking too much" or worrying too much. A lack of support from a woman's partner or financial concerns can lead to this *toas*. The primary symptom was weight loss, but Khmer women also mentioned poor appetite and weakness. Anger, frustration, and unhappiness were commonly reported emotional symptoms. "Acting crazy" also occurred in some women. Mothers considered *pruey cet* to be an especially serious *toas* that some mothers can die from. Women believed that this postpartum complication is untreatable, or even if it can be treated, it cannot be completely cured.

Phenomenology of Postpartum Depression

In my grounded theory study (Beck, 1993), I discovered that loss of control was the basic social psychologic problem in postpartum depression. Women lacked control over their emotions, thought processes, and actions. Women suffering from postpartum depression attempted to cope with the problem of loss of control through a four-stage process called teetering on the edge, which refers to walking the fine line between sanity and insanity (Figure 5.1). The stages included (1) encountering terror, (2) dying of self, (3) struggling to survive, and (4) regaining control.

Encountering Terror

"In the initial stage, women were hit suddenly and unexpectedly by the postpartum depression. The syndrome can begin within the first few weeks after delivery or can be delayed until 6 months or more after birth.

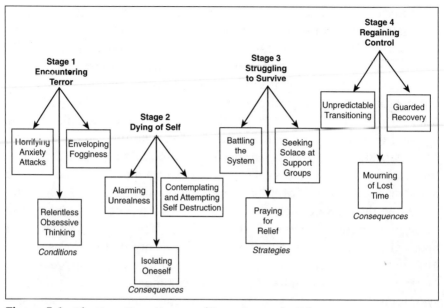

Figure 5.1 The Four-Stage Process of Teetering on the Edge
Reprinted with permission from Beck (1993).

When postpartum depression hit, mothers felt trapped in a dark tunnel with no foreseeable escape. As one mother poignantly described,

> I was on cloud nine through my whole pregnancy. I was very happy in the hospital. Then it hit me when my baby was 14 days old. One night I had my first severe panic attack. I felt like everything was closing in on me. Something just snapped in me, and there was no going back.

Mothers described this onslaught as "going to the gate of hell and back," "your worst possible nightmare," "everything was falling apart piece by piece," "the bottom fell out," and "your whole world turned upside down." Three conditions of encountering terror can occur during this first stage: horrifying anxiety attacks, relentless obsessive thinking, and enveloping fogginess.

> When it first hit me at 7 months, I had a major anxiety attack. It came out of the blue. I just felt numb all over, and I started to hyperventilate. I felt this pain in my chest, so I started to think, "Oh my God, I'm having a heart attack. I'm dying!" It was that every

nerve in my body was exploding—like little fireworks were going off all over my body. I felt like I was going crazy. My skin felt like it was literally crawling. I wished I could rip it off and put it in another body. I would try and wipe my skin off.

Relentless obsessive thinking.

Throughout their waking hours, the women were bombarded with obsessive thoughts, such as these shared by two mothers:

My mothers were extremely obsessive. They would never stop. I thought, "Oh my God, am I going crazy? What if I have to be admitted to the hospital?" And so on. It was just nonstop. I was living constantly in these terrible thoughts that I was a horrible person, a horrible mother, and questioning what is wrong with me. I was just obsessed with this all day long.

Obsessive thinking left the mothers mentally and physically exhausted. At the end of the day, the women could not even look forward to some relief because, as one mother put it, "I would lay in bed and the thoughts would just go and go. I thought I was going to go insane."

Enveloping fogginess.

During this initial stage of postpartum depression, the fogginess settled in. Mothers experienced a loss of concentration and sometimes motor skills. This fogginess is clearly illustrated in the following two quotes from mothers:

I could not concentrate to read a book. I had been a very avid reader and could comprehend well. I lost all that in my postpartum depression. I would have to read lines over two and three times. People would talk to me, and all I would see was their lips moving. Oh, I tried to do something—go out for a run, visit a friend, or take the baby to the mall—but it didn't work. The fogginess would set in.

Dying of Self

As a result of the conditions in the initial stage of postpartum depression, the dying of mothers' normal selves occurred during stage 2. This stage consisted of the following three consequences: alarming unrealness, isolating oneself, and contemplating and attempting self-destruction. These three consequences were involuntary responses to the conditions in stage 1.

Alarming unrealness.

In alarming unrealness, mothers' normal selves were no longer present. Neither the women nor their husbands knew who these women were. Husbands asked where their wives had gone. During postpartum depression, women repeatedly said that they did not feel real. They felt like robots just going through motions of taking care of their babies. They felt void and empty of any caring emotions. Several mothers vividly described this transformation:

> *One minute I'd be socializing. All of a sudden, it would feel like all of those emotions were being sucked away from you and you'd go back into that void of a robot, like you'd just start acting. It's very scary. You feel as though you are not the same person. You are afraid your children aren't going to have you for a mother. The roughest part was between my husband and me. It had gotten to the point where I didn't know him anymore because he didn't know me anymore. He felt like he was living with a Dr. Jekyll and Mr. Hyde. My big fear was that I wasn't going to ever be the person I had been before postpartum depression. It was terrifying, and I'd cry hysterically.*

Isolating oneself.

Isolation was another consequence of the second stage of postpartum depression. Mothers lost all interest in things that they had previously enjoyed, their interests and goals, and their families and friends. They felt alienated and alone because they believed that no one understood what they were going through. They feared that people thought they were bad mothers. Some of the women isolated themselves in their homes because they were afraid to go anywhere. They repeatedly expressed a lack of interest in sex. They also experienced a distancing of themselves from their babies:

> *I had these really weird feelings towards my baby. I couldn't be around him. He gave me anxiety, as if he were something bad. I couldn't walk past the door of his room without being anxious.*

Contemplating and attempting self-destruction.

A third consequence of the first stage of encountering terror was contemplating and attempting self-destruction. Not only were these mothers pondering death, but some also attempted self-destruction. Contributing to their thoughts of death was the guilt they carried because of their perceptions of being failures as mothers and to their thoughts of harming their babies:

> I would go into my baby's room and think, "Put the blanket over his head. He's nothing." Then I'd start crying hysterically. I felt like the worst person in the world, the worst mother in the world. I felt tremendous guilt and just wanted to hurt myself.

> I started thinking death thoughts at one point. I didn't plan suicide, but I started thinking that I'd be better off dead. I had never been that low in my whole life when I thought death was the way to go. I just wanted to get out of this world. It was like everything was black.

Two women not only contemplated self-destruction but also attempted to carry out these thoughts by overdosing or cutting their wrists.

Struggling to Survive

In struggling to survive, the third stage of teetering on the edge, women employed the following three strategies: battling the system, praying for relief, and seeking solace in a postpartum depression support group. The consequences in stage two became conditions requiring strategies by the women. Consequences of one set of actions can become part of the conditions affecting the next set of actions occurring in a sequence (Strauss & Corbin, 1990).

Battling the system.
After the decision had been made to seek professional help, women began a tortuous path to find the appropriate treatment. Mothers experience disappointment, frustration, humiliation, and anger in their initial call to health professionals for help:

> I picked up my phone and called my obstetrician. He never returned the phone call. Three days later I called again, and he told me there's nothing he could do for me and not to waste my time coming there just to talk.

> I was very, very disappointed in my obstetrician's response to me. He patted me on the back and was very patronizing and said, "You are only a mild case. I've had women come in here who were 10 times worse.

Obstetricians gave women the names and numbers of psychiatrists. However, some of these referrals were not successful, as not all psychiatrists were knowledgeable about postpartum depression. The search would have to continue until a knowledgeable psychiatrist was found.

The use of antidepressants was the treatment of choice by psychiatrists, and Prozac was the drug prescribed most often. Some mothers required shock therapy and psychiatric hospitalization in addition to medications.

During their postpartum depression, some mothers found that they began to become hypochondriacs and reported physical symptoms. Some experienced chest pains during anxiety attacks and often went to the emergency room to validate that they were not having a heart attack.

Finances hindered some mothers from obtaining the professional help that they needed, and health insurance often did not adequately cover the costs of psychiatric care.

> We couldn't afford to see a regular psychiatrist at over $100 an
> hour. We just didn't have that kind of money. So I went to our
> church for counseling, but they weren't really equipped to help me
> with my postpartum depression.

Praying for relief.
In addition to battling the system, women turned to prayer as a strategy in their struggle to survive:

> The Lord was what really got me through a lot. It was just a lot of
> prayer and crying to the Lord that helped me get through it. I used
> to go to church and pray for hours. My God, how much more can I
> endure! You're not a vindictive or hateful God, but why is this hap-
> pening to me? You have to get me out of this because I cannot take
> this any longer.

Seeking a solace in a support group.
Attending a postpartum depression support group was the third strategy that women used in their struggle to survive. The support group helped to counter the isolation and loneliness the mothers felt while introducing them to women who had recovered from postpartum depression. It provided hope that their depression could be overcome and that they would regain control of their lives again. Being among other women suffering from postpartum depression helped to confirm the reality of the

condition for the mothers. One woman poignantly described the benefits that she received from the group:

> *My doctor never told me about other women with postpartum depression. I was in the total dark the whole time. It wasn't until I started coming to the support group that I realized, for God's sake, that other women went through this!*

Regaining Control

Regaining control was the fourth and final stage in the substantive theory of teetering on the edge. Regaining control was a slow process consisting of three consequences: unpredictable transitioning, mourning lost time, and guarded recovering.

Unpredictable transitioning.

The process of recovery from postpartum depression was not sudden. Occasionally, among the bad days, there would be a good one. Gradually, the number of good days experienced would increase until only a few bad days cropped up here and there. These would be unpredictable. This erratic transition to regaining control is illustrated in the following quote:

> *When I got out of my severest depression, I had more good times than bad times. I had days where I felt like nothing had ever happened. I mean I was normal. I really felt such intense love for my baby. I could have a relationship with my husband. Then the next day for no reason at all I'd wake up and just be off.*

Mourning lost time.

As the mothers progressed in their recovery from postpartum depression, they began to mourn the lost time that they would not be able to recapture with their infants:

> *I feel robbed of the first 6 months of my daughter's life. I never really got to hold her as a baby, and I feel cheated.*

Another mother repeatedly walked through the baby departments of stores in the mall looking at infant clothes, mourning that her baby's infancy that had been lost because of postpartum depression. Throughout the recovery period, the mothers needed to work through these feelings of being cheated of the opportunity to experience unique periods of their children's lives.

Guarded recovery.

Guarded recovery was the final consequence of the strategies of struggling to survive. This occurred when the mothers felt they had essentially recovered from postpartum depression. Mothers repeatedly noted how at this point in their recovery their husbands would say, "Thank God, my wife is finally back!" When mothers felt better, they would talk about how all of the symptoms of postpartum depression just eventually faded away:

> When I was sick, I didn't want my baby. I didn't love my husband. I didn't want to work. I hated everything. When I got better, it all melted away.

Postpartum depression, however, left an indelible mark on mothers' lives. Even after regaining control, they repeatedly stated that they still feared that at some point in the future they could be stricken with the depression again.

> Postpartum depression makes you very, very vulnerable. You still feel like you're on a fine line between sanity and insanity because when it first happened it came out of nowhere. You're normal and then next thing you know you're crazy.

Reprinted with permission from Beck, Teetering on the edge: A substantive theory of postpartum depression. *Nursing Research*, 42, pp. 44–47 (1993).

Postpartum Depression: A Metasynthesis

Despite the fact that qualitative studies on postpartum depression have increased in numbers, clinical application and knowledge development will be hindered unless the powerful findings from these studies are synthesized through a metasynthesis. A metasynthesis refers to overarching generalizations that can result from integrating and comparing results from individual qualitative studies (Sandelowski, Docherty, & Emden, 1997).

I (Beck, 2002) conducted a metasynthesis of 18 qualitative studies that I had located in the literature. It was my hope that by enlarging the interpretive possibilities of the findings from these 18 individual qualitative studies that a larger narrative on mothers' experiences with postpartum depression would provide a greater impact on direction for clinical practice if they were placed in a larger interpretive context.

These 18 studies were conducted in various countries in the world. Eight studies were conducted in the United Kingdom, six in the United States, three in Australia, and one in Canada. Integrating these studies into a whole that was more than each of the individual studies yielded four overarching themes or perspectives involved with postpartum depression: (1) incongruity between expectations and reality of motherhood, (2) spiraling downward, (3) pervasive loss, and (4) making gains (Figure 5.2). As shown in Figure 5.2, women can move back and forth between these four perspectives, and they can be in more than one at any time.

The results of this metasynthesis of postpartum depression provide implications for clinical practice. Examples of two such implications can be derived from the overarching themes of (1) incongruity between expectations and the reality of motherhood and (2) pervasive loss.

The women's unrealistic expectations of motherhood were shattered by the reality of their own lives as new mothers. These conflicting expectations and experiences of motherhood resulted in their becoming overwhelmed, perceiving themselves as failures as mothers, and bearing a suffocating burden of guilt. Clinicians have a responsibility to take an active role in stopping the harmful myths of motherhood that are so prevalent in our society and that put our mothers' mental health at risk.

Loss emerged as a pervasive component of this postpartum mood disorder. The types of losses identified in this metasynthesis can help health care providers differentiate the many kinds of loss that mothers may be grappling with. Jeanne in 1990 proposed the use of loss and grief frameworks to

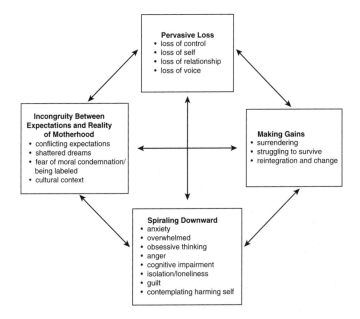

Figure 5.2 Four Perspectives of Postpartum Depression.
Reprinted with permission from Beck, Postpartum depression: A metasynthesis. *Qualitative Health Research*, 12, p. 461 (2002).

explain postpartum depression (Driscoll, 1990). The findings of this meta-synthesis confirm Jeanne's framework as a key model for clinicians to use in developing interventions for postpartum depressed mothers. Giving birth to a baby is universally viewed as a gain rather than a loss. Loss must first be identified as such before the healing grief work can start. As a postpartum depressed mother puts her losses into perspective, she can then move into the final stage of grief work, which is healing and restoration.

Postpartum Depressive Symptomatology in Adolescents

Adolescent mothers are not immune to postpartum depression. In a review of maternal health data, as many as 48% of 1,000 adolescent mothers reported experiencing depressive symptoms (Deal & Holt, 1998). Elevated levels of depressive symptoms have been identified in 47% of adolescents during the postpartum period (Barnet, Joffe, Duggan, Wilson, & Repke, 1996; Miller, 1998). One possible reason for this high rate is the overwhelming demands of new motherhood and adolescence plus low levels of support (Logsdon, 2004).

To help clinicians understand adolescent mothers' depressive symptoms better after the birth of their infants, Clemmens (2002) conducted a qualitative study of 20 adolescent mothers between the ages of 16 and 18 years. From in-depth interviews, six themes emerged: (1) suddenly realizing motherhood and feeling scared because there was nothing that these adolescent mothers could do to change this, (2) being pulled and torn between the responsibilities of adolescence and motherhood, (3) constantly questioning and trying to understand their depressive symptoms and what was happening to them, (4) feeling alone, betrayed, and rejected by their peers and family, (5) feeling like everything was falling down on them, and (6) feeling like they were changing and regrouping for a different future.

Postpartum Depression in Adoptive Mothers

Postpartum disorders can occur in women who adopt children. For many of these women, there is a history of infertility. Some have taken various medications to promote fertility and have experienced the stressors of not conceiving a child. Conceiving and then experiencing a miscarriage(s) were the experiences of other women. These events cause a significant amount of brain strain on each woman's biology. This is a population of women that will not be screened in the obstetrical offices or by the ante-natal professionals. Thus, it is imperative for pediatric providers, family practitioners, adoption agencies, and early intervention programs to be on the look out for these women in distress.

It is doubtful that women experiencing difficulty after the adoption of a child are going to come forth and seek help. The social context is more one of "you got what you wanted, so now what is wrong?" These women may struggle in silence, constantly asking themselves why they are feeling bad, as they finally have the baby/child that they hoped for. It is imperative that pediatricians and family practice providers be cognizant of the impact of adoption on the woman and her family. The new mother is experiencing anxiety, stress, disrupted sleep, role changes, role adjustments, issues of integration into the community of other mothers, and redefining her self and her way of being in the world. Continuous assessment as to how she is doing is mandatory.

In 1952, Victoroff described postpartum depression in three adoptive mothers. Melges (1968) also reported depression in three new mothers after having adopted infants. VanPutten and LaWall (1981) described post-partum depression and psychosis in adoptive mothers. Bond (1995) first coined the term postadoption depression syndrome.

Gair (1999) interviewed 19 adoptive mothers of babies and young children up to 5 years of age. The majority of children of the adoptive mothers were between 5 to 9 weeks old at the time of the adoption. Mothers also completed the EPDS. Gair reported that six mothers (32%) scores on the EPDS indicated high levels of postpartum depressive symptoms. Gair concluded from her interviews and the EPDS responses that some adoptive mothers do experience depression as a result of the arrival of a new infant into their lives as evidenced by one mother's comments: "*You can write this in big letters,* ADOPTIVE MOTHERS CAN GET POSTNATAL DEPRESSION, *and it's not just me, others have said the same"* (1999, p. 62).

Foli and Thompson (2004) interviewed dozens of parents about their postadoption experiences and here are some of their responses: "I was chronically sad." "I felt panicked, total fear." "I gained 30 pounds." "I couldn't sleep." "The guilt was horrible." "I didn't know what to do." "I paced back and forth." "I stopped eating. That never happens to me." "I felt melancholy." "I didn't feel depressed, but I felt a lot of anxiety." "I felt angry" (p. 191).

Foli and Thompson (2004) concluded that their research identified that postpartum depression and postadoption depression share some of the same underlying themes. The adoptive parents who were interviewed by Foli and Thompson reported experiences in six of the seven dimensions of symptoms assessed by the Postpartum Depression Screening Scale (Beck & Gable, 2002) (see Chapter 9). The one category of symptoms not reported by the adoptive parents was thoughts of harming themselves. Foli and Thompson stated, however, that this was not a question that they had asked of adoptive parents in their research. Foli and Thompson found that the onset of postadoption depression can occur years after the adoption has taken place and lasts for years.

McCarthy (2000) conducted an exploratory study with parents from the eastern European adoptive community by an online survey. The Internet sample of parents who adopted children internationally consisted of 145 respondents. Of the 145 respondents, 65% reported experiencing postadoption depression. McCarthy found through her research that postadoption depression is not dependent on the age of the child when adopted.

Postpartum Depression in Pregnancy Loss

Research has consistently shown that women who experience a pregnancy loss report a higher level of depressive symptoms and a higher incidence of postpartum depression than women who have given birth to a living baby. In the early period after miscarriage, 22% to 44% of women experience significant depressive levels (Jackman, McGee, & Turner, 1991; Neugebauer, Kline, & O'Connor, 1992; Prettyman, Cordle, & Cook, 1993; Thapar & Thapar, 1992).

Janssen, Cuisinier, Hoogduin, and deGraauw (1996) conducted a prospective longitudinal study comparing depressive symptoms in 227 women who had lost their babies and 213 women who had given birth to a living baby over a period of 18 months. At 6 months after pregnancy loss, women who had experienced a loss reported significantly higher levels of depressive symptoms than women who had not experienced such a loss. By 12 to 18 months, the depressive levels of women who had miscarried improved, and there was no longer a significant difference between the two groups of women.

A smaller number of studies have used structured clinical interviews to determine the prevalence of postpartum depression and not just measured depressive levels. Early studies reported that 1 to 3 months after miscarriage 48% to 51% of the women were clinically depressed (Friedman & Gath, 1989; Garel, Blondel, Lelong, Papin Bonenfant & Kaminski1992). In Hong Kong, Lee et al. (1997), using the Structured Clinical Interview for DSM-IV Axis 1 Disorders (SCID), interviewed 156 women at 6 weeks and reported that 16 women (10.3%) met the DSM-III-R criteria for major depression.

Swanson (2000) tested a path model based on Lazarus' theory of emotions and adaptation for predicting the intensity of women's depressive symptoms at 4 months and 1 year after miscarriage. The sample was composed of 174 women who had experienced a miscarriage before 20-weeks gestation. This model accounted for 63% and 54% of the variance in women's depressive symptoms at 4 months and 1 year, respectively. Women at the highest risk for depressive symptoms after miscarriage are women who attribute high personal significance to the pregnancy loss, have low levels of social support, have low emotional strength, use passive coping strategies, have a low income, and do not conceive or give birth by 1 year after miscarriage.

Postpartum Depressive Symptoms in Fathers

Over the first year after delivery, the rate of postpartum depression symptoms in fathers has ranged from 10.1% (Matthey et al., 2000) to 28.6% (Areias, Kumar, Barras, & Figueiredo, 1996) in the community-based samples. When focusing on men whose spouses had postpartum depression, the rates of paternal depression ranged from 24% (Zelkowitz & Milet, 2001) to 50% (Lovestone & Kumar, 1993). Research is finding that the onset of fathers' depression occurs later in the postpartum period than the onset of depression in mothers (Matthey et al., 2000).

Significant predictors of elevated postpartum depressive symptoms in fathers include depression in spouses, either during the prenatal or postpartum period (Areias et al., 1996; Zelkowitz & Milet, 2001), a personal history of depression, and the couples' relationship and functioning (Matthey et al., 2000). Postpartum depression in mothers is significantly correlated with depression in fathers (Deater-Deckard, Pickering, Dunn, & Golding, 1998; Dudley, Roy, Kelk, & Bernard, 2001). Fathers were significantly more likely to experience postpartum depressive symptoms if their partner/spouse had postpartum depression.

In two qualitative studies, the fathers' experiences of living with a partner suffering from postpartum depression were examined (Boath, Pryce, & Cox, 1998; Meignan, Davis, Thomas, & Droppleman, 1999). Fathers expressed an array of negative emotions such as confusion, fear, anger, helplessness, and frustration. The fathers were concerned for their partner, their disrupted family life, financial problems, and uncertainty regarding the future.

Cheryl's meta-analyses have revealed the significant negative impact of postpartum depression on mother–infant interaction and child development (Beck, 1995, 1998). If both the mother and the father are experiencing postpartum depression or elevated depressive symptoms, this combination may further add to the risk of their children's development (Deater-Deckard et al., 1998).

A group program for women who are suffering from postpartum depression and their partners was conducted with one of the eight sessions focusing on the couple (Morgan, Matthey, Barnett, & Richardson, 1997). Concerns of the men focused on their frustration of trying to help their partners but not being appreciated for their assistance. The help that men tried to provide their partners can be divided into instrumental support and emotional support. When providing instrumental support, the men found it rejected by their partners. The women were critical of their efforts to help. Regarding their attempts to give emotional support to their postpartum depressed partners, the fathers shared that no matter how hard they tried, they could not please their partner.

Postpartum Depressed Mothers' Experiences in Interacting with Their Children

In my research, I (Cheryl) conducted a qualitative study with 12 postpartum depressed mothers to explore their experiences caring for and interacting with their infants and older children (Beck, 1996c). From in-depth interviews with these mothers, nine themes emerged.

"Theme 1: Postpartum depression overtook mothers' minds and bodies, preventing them from reaching out to their infants and depriving them of any feelings of joy.

"Mothers vividly described postpartum depression as something physically overtaking them and possessing their minds and bodies. Even if mothers wanted to reach out to their infants, they could not control their behavior. One primipara painfully stated, "I had no control of my own self-being, nothing, mind, soul, nothing. It basically controlled me. I wanted to reach out to my baby, yet I couldn't."

Pleasure and enjoyment were not experienced as components of the maternal care-taking role:

> *I'd look at the new baby and think he was a beautiful baby. I'd try to focus on that because I love children, but that real deep joy that you have wasn't there. I could not enjoy holding the baby or taking care of him. I just felt like the postpartum depression was taking the total joy out of the baby.*

When caring for their infants, postpartum depressed mothers repeatedly expressed how mechanical they felt. Women would joylessly go through the motions of feeding their infants, changing diapers, and caring for them: "I just went through the motions making sure my baby was fed. I was just like a robot. I would pick her up. I would breastfeed her. I would put her down. I was just walking around the house like a zombie." Contributing to their robotic image of themselves as mothers was the occasional feeling of not being real, as if someone had drugged them:

> *It's like you're just not real. You're there and you're not there with the baby. It wasn't even occurring to me that it was my baby—this thing, it was mine.*

Theme 2: Overwhelmed by the responsibilities for caring for their children, the women were petrified that they would not be able to cope.

For postpartum depressed mothers, the responsibility for childcare seemed absolutely enormous. Mothers continually questioned their ability to cope adequately with the increasing demands of their infants and older children. Previously confident, independent women were reduced to pleading with their husbands not to go to work and leave them alone to interact with their children, as illustrated in the two following situations:

> *After a week and a half my husband had to go back to work. I started crying and said to him, "Oh my God, I can't be alone with two kids." I was so afraid because I knew that I was upset a lot. I said, "Oh my God, I am going to be upset, and I am going to be home alone."*

> *Every time my baby cried when she woke up, I'd feel a chill go up my body, and I wanted her to stay asleep because I knew it was so hard when she woke up. The fear of the baby needing you or crying for your help. . . .*

Other women surrounded themselves with family and friends throughout the day so that they would not be alone with their babies. The thought of being home alone with their infants terrified some mothers.

Theme 3: To survive, some mothers erected a wall to separate themselves emotionally and physically from their children.

At times, mothers had to separate themselves physically from the constant demands being placed on them from their children. What little energy they had left was being drained. One postpartum depressed mother and her infant were fortunate enough to be living temporarily with a relative who could step in and care for the infant when the mother had to separate herself:

> I went to live at my mom's. It was a two-family house. The attic was done over. I lived upstairs in the attic. I would come down and get as much motherhood as I could and then went back up to the attic.

Theme 4: Stripped of a strong desire to interact with their children and plagued by oversensitivity to stimuli, mothers often failed to respond to their infants' cues.

When suffering through postpartum depression, mothers did not yearn to interact with their infants and did not reciprocate their babies' smiles and sounds. As one mother disclosed,

> The baby was smiling and cooing at me, and I was just looking at her, not smiling or cooing back, not interacting with her, not getting her to go further. I just stared at her saying, "Why am I not smiling back at this baby who is happy-go-lucky and has been sleeping through the night since 2 weeks?"

Another factor contributing to some women's lack of response to their infants' cues was their oversensitivity to noise, light, and other stimuli. Sounds and light were perceived as being magnified so much that at times some mothers tried to block these stimuli:

> My son's sounds were incredibly loud, which means that everything was magnified so that ordinary speech sounded like you were shouting at me. Light was also very bright. All my perceptions were up, so outside stimuli were being received in some funny way.

Theme 5: Guilt and irrational thinking pervaded mothers' minds during their day-to-day interactions with their children.

Postpartum depressed mothers perceived themselves as being the worst mothers in the world. They were filled with pain-ridden guilt for not being able to love their babies as they thought they should. One mother described her guilt:

> *The fact that I couldn't love her normally made the guilt even worse.*
> *You just don't feel anything good for your baby. You just feel full of*
> *guilt. One night I actually remember walking in the room and*
> *looking at her sleeping in the crib. I was crying because I felt so bad*
> *for her that I was her mother.*

Mothers were haunted by the effects of their depressive behavior on their infants and older children. One woman, a multipara, recounted this:

> *I remember when she was about 6 months old holding her in my*
> *psychiatrist's office. I had started to cry, and my psychiatrist noticed*
> *it.[The baby] reached up and stroked my face, and that made me*
> *very happy but also very sad and guilty because I really didn't*
> *think that she should have to feel responsible for comforting me. It*
> *became very clear that it was really a big burden to put on kids if*
> *they have to feel they have that kind of responsibility.*

Irrational thinking also plagued some mothers as they interacted with their children. One mother described the following incident:

> *For me, what was out of control and still is to this day is the irra-*
> *tional thoughts that keep racing through my mind as I care for my*
> *baby. I would be going along and being okay, and then I would get*
> *up to that changing table and in a matter of seconds my mind would*
> *have started with, "Oh, the baby is going to fall of the table. I don't*
> *care if she falls off the table." Why did I think that I don't care if she*
> *falls of the table? Of course I care.*

Theme 6: Uncontrollable anger erupted periodically toward the children to the degree that mothers feared that they might harm their children.

For many women, uncontrollable anger was a new and distressing emotion for them. For the first time in their lives, some women were terrified that at some point their anger would erupt to such a degree that they could hurt their children, as in the following situation:

> *I would get real angry. It's really scary because you've heard these*
> *stories about mothers being in court for smothering their baby and*
> *my first thought was fry the woman. I mean, can you believe they'd*
> *do that to a helpless child? And to be able to understand that!*

When their anger started to flare up, mothers would put distance between themselves and their children to ensure their safety. For some mothers, this uncontrollable anger toward their children was the deciding factor that drove them to seeking professional help.

Theme 7: As postpartum depression engulfed the mothers, they perceived that detrimental relationships with their older children were materializing.

As a result of their inability to cope with more than one child at a time, mothers resented their older children and pushed them away. Mothers felt as if the older children were suffocating them when they tried to vie for attention. One mother noted this:

> When I was going through the depression really bad, I pushed away
> my daughter and my husband. It was like I just wanted to take care
> of the baby and I didn't want to take care of anyone else. I could
> only deal with one person, and the rest of you should go away,
> because I can't deal with the rest of it.

When struggling through postpartum depression, mothers forced themselves to provide for the basic needs of their older children, but anything beyond that was an impossibility. One mother revealed that once her older son was bathed, fed, and dressed, she plopped him down in front of the television for the rest of the morning so that she would not have to deal with him.

Mothers perceived that as a result of their postpartum depression, their older children became confused and began to act out to gain their mothers' attention. The following quote reveals some of the repercussions of postpartum depression on older children in the family:

> If my 6-year-old daughter was acting up, I'd say to her, "Why are
> you acting like this?" My daughter said, "At least you yell at me.
> It's better than you not paying any attention to me at all." And I
> thought, "My God!"

Theme 8: Feelings of loss enveloped the mothers as they dwelled on their relationships with their children.

Postpartum depression was viewed as a thief, robbing mothers of the intimacy with their children. One primipara prayed to God that she would not have postpartum depression a second time because she felt so cheated of the first 3 to 4 months of her baby's life. The residual pain of this loss did not lessen even with the birth of a second child.

Women grieved over the lost relationship with their children as any sense of normalcy in the coveted role as mother was lost. Some women were tormented about how their children would suffer if they did not recover. One said this:

> You don't want your children just in good hands. You want your fingerprints on their lives.

Theme 9: Striving to minimize the negative effects of postpartum depression on their children, mothers attempted to put their children's needs above their own.

Making sure their children were being well taken care of was the first priority of mothers, even when they were feeling horrible. As one mother stated,

> Even though my emotions were so out of control with postpartum depression, it didn't get in the way of me taking care of my baby, which was the number one thing now in my life, to take care of this child that was so totally helpless.

At times, mothers forced themselves to interact with and smile at their infants in attempts to protect them from the ill effects of postpartum depression. The following passage describes a mother's placing her infant's needs above her own:

> I thought about [taking] a razor blade to my wrists every day during the worst of my depression; well, if it weren't for my son— you see, my maternal instincts never left. I felt like, God, this poor child growing up knowing his mother killed herself because of him. That was the biggest thing that kept me from doing it.

Mothering by proxy was urged by the women to ensure that the babies would not be deprived of love. Grandmothers, sisters, and friends were enlisted to help hold, cuddle, and interact with the babies. Another protective measure taken by some women was shielding infants and older children from seeing their mothers crying. When mothers started crying, they would leave the room their children were in. Some mothers enrolled older children in play groups to counteract the decreased stimulation that they were receiving at home."

Reprinted with permission from Beck, Postpartum depressed mothers' experiences interacting with their children. Nursing Research, 45, 100–103, 1996.

The Effects of Postpartum Depression on Maternal–Infant Interaction

Evidence is mounting that indicates postpartum depression negatively affects mother–infant interactions. Because the mother most often constitutes the newborn's main social environment during the first months of the rapidly developing infant, these findings are of special concern. Infants are extremely sensitive to the quality of their interpersonal environment.

Since the 1980s, Field's research program has consistently found that maternal depression negatively affects infants as early as the neonatal period. The infants experience disorganizing effects of their depressed mothers' interaction behavior. Field (1998) described the dysregulation profile of infants of depressed mothers. These infants have decreased responsivity on the Brazelton, increased indeterminate sleep, and increased levels of norepinephrine and cortisol during the neonatal period, right frontal electroencephalogram (EEG) activation, decreased responsivity to facial expressions, decreased vagal tone, symptoms of neurologic delays at 6 months, decreased play and exploratory behavior, low Bayley mental and motor scale scores, and lower weight percentiles by 12 months of age (Field, Fox, Pickens, Nawrocki, & Soutullo, 1995).

Compared with nondepressed mothers, postpartum depressed mothers displayed less affectionate contact behavior with their infants, were less responsive to their infants' cues, and were withdrawn with flatness of affect or were hostile and intrusive. Infants of depressed mothers tend to be fussier and more discontent, avoidant, and make fewer positive facial expressions and vocalizations with their mothers compared with infants of nondepressed women.

In the United Kingdom, Murray, Fiori-Cowley, Hooper, and Cooper (1996a) also reported similar findings at 2 months after delivery. Depressed mothers interacted significantly less sensitively, more rejecting, and less affirming with their infants. Infants of postpartum depressed mothers were more likely to display abrupt breaks in their attention and engagement compared with infants whose mothers were not depressed. Murray et al. also found that the insensitive mothers precipitated these disruptions in their infants' attention and behavior.

Another recent study conducted in Switzerland again confirmed the results of Field's (1998) and Murray and Cooper's (1997) programs of research. Righetti-Veltema, Conne-Perreard, Bousquet, and Manzano (2002) reported that at 3 months after delivery, deleterious effects of postpartum depression on mother–infant relationships were apparent. The depressed mother–infant dyads were less vocal, had fewer visual communications, smiled less, and had fewer corporal interactions than nondepressed mother–infant pairs.

Kaplan, Bachorowski, Smoski, and Hudenko (2002) demonstrated how a specific infant learning process is adversely affected by postpartum depression. By comparing examined recorded speech segments between postpartum depressed mother–infant dyads, Kaplan et al. discovered that the infants displayed no sign of associative learning in respect to their mother's speech but did learn to respond readily to an unfamiliar nondepressed mother's speech.

Touch behavior and content of child-directed speech were examined in 72 mothers and their infants during play. Eighteen depressed mother–infant pairs and 18 control pairs were observed when the infants were 6 months old. Also, 18 more depressed mothers and their infants were observed when those infants were 10 months old. Postpartum depressive symptoms were measured by the EPDS. Compared with nondepressed mothers, depressed women lifted their infants with more restraining behaviors. Depressed mothers used less affective and informative features in their speech compared with nondepressed women. Infants of depressed mothers spent more time touching themselves rather than their mothers or a toy. The authors perceived this infant behavior as compensating for the lack of positive touching from their mothers.

Cheryl conducted a meta-analysis of 19 studies that investigated the effects of postpartum depression on mother–infant interaction during the first year of life (Beck, 1995). I examined the magnitude of the following three subcategories of maternal–infant interaction: maternal interactive behavior, infant interactive behavior, and dyadic interactive behavior (interaction patterns or shared states between mothers and their infants). Analysis revealed that postpartum depression had a moderate adverse effect on both maternal and infant interactive behavior and a large negative effect on dyadic interactive behavior. If a woman is emotionally unavailable or unresponsive affectively, synchrony of interactive behaviors is unlikely to take place in depressed mother–infant pairs. Depressed mothers may fail to pick up on their infants' cries and smiles.

In a community sample of 72 primiparous depressed mothers and 50 nondepressed mothers at 2 to 3 months postpartum, the effect of postpartum depression on mother–infant interactions, infant response to the still-face perturbation, and performance on an instrumental learning task were assessed (Stanley, Murray, & Stern, 2004). Compared with nondepressed mothers, postpartum depressed mothers showed significantly lower rates of positive contingent responsiveness and higher rates of negative contingent responsiveness to their infants. No adverse effects of postpartum depression were found on the infants' performance on still-face infant perturbation or on the instrumental learning task.

Clinical trials are needed to determine the most effective early intervention programs for postpartum depressed mothers and its adverse disruptions to the mother–infant pairs. Field described four effective interventions. First is massage therapy for infants. Field et al. (1996) reported that infants who are born to depressed adolescent mothers and who experience massage therapy for 15 minutes for 2 days a week over a 6-week period cried less and spent more time in active alert and active awake states than the control group of infants who were rocked in rocking chairs. The massage therapy infants also gained more weight and displayed greater improvement in their sociability and soothability than the control group of infants (Pickens & Field, 1993).

Mood-induction interventions for postpartum depressed mothers are the second type of suggested intervention (Field et al., 1996). As short-term interventions, massage therapy and music therapy just before a mother–infant interaction can be used to alter the depressed mother's mood state, if only for the length of time of her immediate interactions with her infant.

In the third approach, interactive coaching, the depressed mother tries to get her infant's attention and imitates all of her infant's behaviors during a face-to-face interaction. When attempting to obtain their infants' attention, mothers were more animated, and mothers' sensitivity to their infants was increased as they imitated their infants' behaviors. Finally, Field et al. viewed nondepressed fathers as buffers for the infants against postpartum depressed mothers' nonempathetic behavior styles of passive/withdrawn and angry/aggressive.

Impact of Postpartum Depression on Children's Cognitive Development and Emotional Behavior

Does postpartum depression result in long-term sequelae for children whose mothers had suffered from this mood disorder? Some longitudinal studies are being conducted to answer this important question, especially by the research teams of Murray et al. (1999) and Hay, Pawlby, Angold, Harold, and Sharp (2003).

First, focusing on cognitive development, in the United Kingdom, Murray et al. (1996a) reported that at 18 months old, boys of postpartum depressed mothers performed significantly poorer on the Bayley Scales of Infant Mental Development (Bayley, 1969) than boys whose mothers had not experienced postpartum depression. There was not a significant effect for girls.

In Switzerland, Righetti-Veltema, Bousquet, and Manzano (2003) examined the impact of postpartum depressive symptoms at 3 months after delivery on the cognitive development of the children 15 months later. Using the Bayley Scales, the 18-month old infants of postpartum depressed mothers performed significantly lower on object concept tasks compared with a control group of infants of nondepressed mothers.

Murray, Hipwell, Hooper, Stein, and Cooper (1996b) followed the same sample of children (Murray et al., 1996a) for 5 years and retested these children. No relationship was found between postpartum depression and the children's performance on cognitive tasks at 5 years of age. Sharp et al. (1995), on the other hand, followed children of postpartum mothers with depression for 4 years and reported that boys of the postpartum depressed mothers scored significantly lower on the perceptual, motor, and verbal subscales of the McCarthy Scales of Children's Abilities (McCarthy, 1972) than girls or children of mothers who had not experienced postpartum depression.

A prospective, longitudinal study was conducted in Barbados of mothers and infants in which measurements were made at birth, at 7 weeks, at 3- and 6-months postpartum, and again at 11 years old (Galler et al., 2004); maternal mood was measured with the Zung Depression Scale and the Zung Anxiety Scale. The Common Entrance Examination for high school was completed by 169 of the children in the original study. Postpartum depression and anxiety were found to predict lower Common Entrance Examination scores, especially English scores, in these 11 year olds.

The emotional development and behavior of children of postpartum depressed mothers have also been examined. Evidence is mounting that postpartum depression is associated with later problems in the children's emotional and behavioral adjustment. Studies have repeatedly indicated that toddlers whose mothers had suffered from postpartum depression displayed more insecure attachment to their mothers compared with children of nondepressed mothers (Murray et al., 1996a; Righetti-Veltema et al., 2003).

School-age children of postpartum depressed mothers have displayed increased behavior problems when they started school. In two studies, teachers completed questionnaires regarding children's behavior. In one of these studies, children in kindergarten whose mothers had postpartum depression were rated more often by their teachers as displaying higher internalizing symptoms (overanxious and depressed) as well as higher externalizing symptoms (oppositional defiant, overt aggression, and conduct problems) than kindergartners whose mothers had not been depressed during their children's infancy (Essex, Klein, Miech, & Smider, 2001). In their prospective study of 5-year-old children, postpartum depression was significantly associated with increased levels of child disturbance in boys. Boys of postpartum depressed mothers showed significantly more hyperactive behavior and behavioral disturbance (Sinclair & Murray, 1998).

In Finland, mothers' postpartum depressive symptoms predicted low social competence in 8- to 9-year-old children (Luoma et al., 2001). Mothers completed the Child Behavior Checklist (Achenbach, 1991). Children with high externalizing and total problem levels were significantly more likely to have mothers who had suffered from postpartum depression than children of nondepressed mothers. No differences were found in internalizing symptoms.

I (Beck, 1998) conducted a meta-analysis to summarize the research and determine the magnitude of the cumulative adverse effects of living with and being socialized by postpartum depressed mothers during the first year of life on children's cognitive and emotional development. Nine studies were included, and the meta-analysis revealed a small but significant effect of postpartum depression on children's cognitive and emotional development. Children whose mothers had experienced postpartum depression displayed more behavior problems and lower cognitive functioning as compared with children of nondepressed mothers.

One of the longest prospective studies looking at the impact of postpartum depression on children has been conducted in the United Kingdom. Hay et al. (2003) have been following children of mothers who were depressed postpartum for 11 years. Their most recent study had mothers, teachers, and children report on violent symptoms of the children at 11 years old. Violent symptoms included engaging in fights, which involved kicking, punching, biting, and pulling hair. Fighting often resulted in injury and suspension from school. Some children used weapons in their fights such as chains, bricks, and stones. This violent behavior occurred more frequently in boys than in girls. Analysis using structural equation modeling revealed that children's violent behavior was predicted by mothers postpartum depression even when her depression during pregnancy and her later history of depression and family characteristics such as social class and financial crisis were controlled. Violence also included symptoms of attention defiant/hyperactivity disorder and problems with anger management. The children who were reported as most violent had mothers who had been depressed at 3 months postpartum and at least one other time thereafter.

Biological research is beginning to link exposure of infants to postpartum depressed mothers' elevated cortisol levels in their adolescent years (Halligan, Herbert, Goodyer, & Murray, 2004). Early adverse experiences may alter later the hypothalamic–pituitary–adrenal axis, which has been shown to be associated with an increased risk for depression. Elevated morning cortisol levels have predicted the development of depressive disorders in adolescents (Goodyer, Tamplin, Herbert, & Altham, 2000) and adult women (Harris et al., 2000). It was hypothesized that early adversity can increase either the basal secretion of glucocorticoids in later adult life or the reactivity of the hypothalamic–pituitary–adrenal axis to stress.

To investigate the long-term association between children's exposure to postpartum depressive symptoms and their cortisol levels in adolescence, Halligan et al. (2004) measured salivary cortisol levels in two groups of adolescents: 48 adolescents whose mothers had postnatal depression and 39 comparison adolescents whose mothers had not been postnatally depressed. These 13-year-old adolescents were part of a prospective, longitudinal study that began at 2 months postpartum on the development of children of postpartum depressed and well women (Murray, 1992). Morning salivary cortisol levels were significantly higher and more variable in adolescents of postpartum depressed mothers than the comparison adolescents. This cortisol level pattern is one that has been found to predict major depression.

Treatment

Secondary Interventions

The aim of primary prevention is the prevention of postpartum depression. However, after a mother develops this mood disorder, secondary prevention takes center stage. The goal of secondary prevention is to limit the severity of postpartum depression and prevent complications and sequelae. Early diagnosis and prompt treatment are the cornerstones of secondary prevention (Harkness, 1995).

In chapter 9, we address the issue of screening, which is critical for early diagnosis. The focus of this section is on the discussion of secondary prevention strategies that have been reported in the literature. The secondary interventions mainly fall into four categories: support groups, health visitors' interventions, interpersonal psychotherapy (IPT), and massage/relaxation therapy (Table 5.4). In the last column of Table 5.4, the effectiveness of these interventions is reported. After the discussion of these secondary interventions, a section on the psychopharmacologic treatments follows.

Secondary Prevention Strategies: Support Groups

Postpartum support groups described in the literature from different parts of the world have been led by various clinicians, such as health visitors, psychiatrists, psychologists, and nurse researchers. In Canada, two psychologists led social support groups for postpartum depressed mothers (Fleming, Klein & Corter, 1992). Each support group consisted of six to eight mothers with their 6- to 8-week-old infants. These support groups met weekly for 2 hours over an 8-week period. The primary aim of the group was to provide postpartum depressed women with an opportunity to be in contact with other women who are having similar experiences and to share problems and discuss solutions. Different topics were emphasized each week. Weekly topics in sequential order were mothers' pregnancy and delivery experiences, mothers' experiences the first few weeks after delivery, mothers' feelings about motherhood, instruction in infant massage and developmental norms of infants, mothers' concern regarding their changing relationships with their partners, and mothers' feelings about either their return to work or staying at home.

In the United Kingdom, health visitor-led support groups for women suffering from postpartum depression were held weekly for 1 hour and 15 minutes (Pitts, 1995). The goals of the group were to increase women's knowledge of postpartum depression, to discuss expectations of motherhood, to learn relaxation and coping techniques, to learn how to manage anger and to deal with premenstrual tension and stress, to discuss relationships, and to increase assertiveness.

Also in the United Kingdom, Eastwood, Horrocks, and Jones (1995) described the components of their health visitor-initiated support group for postpartum depressed women. Group leaders were health visitors. The support group consisted of five components: confidentiality, counseling, focus on feelings and needs, sharing, and support.

In Taiwan, nurse researcher-led postpartum depression support groups met for four weekly sessions, with each lasting between 1.5 to 2.0 hours

Table 5.4 SECONDARY PREVENTION FOR POSTPARTUM DEPRESSION

POSTPARTUM STUDY/YEAR	INTERVENTION	COUNTRY	SAMPLE SIZE	RESEARCH DESIGN	INSTRUMENT	EFFECT
Cullinan, 1991	Health visitor intervention, six to eight weekly counseling visits	United Kingdom	N = 62 mothers with high EPDS scopes	One group experimental	EPDS	87% of those counseled improved
Fleming et al., 1992	Social support group	Canada	N = 44 EG N = 83 CG N = 15 group-by-mail intervention	Quasi-experimental	Current Experience Scale EPDS MAACL	nonsignificant
Eastwood et al., 1995	Peer group support (health visitor led)	United Kingdom	8	Pre-experimental	EPDS Beck Depression Inventory (BDI) Hospital Anxiety and Depression Scale (HAD)	The severity of symptoms decreased, but no statistics included
Pitts, 1995	Health visitor-led support group	United Kingdom	9	Pre-experimental	EPDS	Seven mothers reduced scores, and two mothers increased their scores

(*continues*)

EG = experimental group
CG = control group

Table 5.4 SECONDARY PREVENTION FOR POSTPARTUM DEPRESSION *(continued)*

POSTPARTUM STUDY/YEAR	INTERVENTION	COUNTRY	SAMPLE SIZE	RESEARCH DESIGN	INSTRUMENT	EFFECT
Field et al., 1996	Massage and relaxation therapy	United States	32 adolescent moms N = 16 massage therapy N = 16 relaxation therapy	Experimental	BDI Profile of Mood States (POMS)	Only massage therapy group experienced a decrease in depression
Stuart and O'Hara, 1995	IPT	United States	N = 6 EG	1 group	BDI Hamilton Rating Scale for Depression	Significant decrease in depressive symptoms
Seeley et al., 1996	Health visitor training	United Kingdom	N = 40 CG N = 40 EG	Quasi-experimental	EPDS	Group of mothers who received the health visitor intervention experienced a 42% decrease in EPDS over 8 weeks
Wickberg and Hwang, 1996	Counseling visits by child health clinic nurses	Sweden	N = 41	Experimental	EPDS MADRS DSM-III-R	Twelve of 15 depressed women (80%) in treatment group showed no evidence of having major depression after receiving six counseling sessions. Only 4 of 15 in the control group (25%) recovered. The difference in recovery rate was significant.

Table 5.4 SECONDARY PREVENTION FOR POSTPARTUM DEPRESSION (*continued*)

POSTPARTUM STUDY/YEAR	INTERVENTION	COUNTRY	SAMPLE SIZE	RESEARCH DESIGN	INSTRUMENT	EFFECT
Meager and Milgrom, 1996	10-week treatment program with educational, social support, and cognitive behavioral components	Australia	N = 10 EG N = 10 CG	Experimental	EPDS BDI POMS	A significant reduction in depression scores
Morgan et al., 1997	Group program for depressed mother and their partners	Australia	34 couples	One group pre–post test	EPDS	A significant decrease in women's scores on EPDS
Chen et al., 2000	Support group	Taiwan	N = 30 EG N = 30 CG	Experimental	BDI	A significant decrease in BDI scores in experimental group
Misri et al., 2000	Partner support	Canada	N = 13 CG N = 16 EG	Experimental	EPDS Mini International Neuropsychiatric Instrument (MINI)	Support group had a significant decrease in depressive symptoms
O'Hara et al., 2000	IPT (12 weeks)	United States	N = 60 EG N = 60 CG	Open treatment trial	Hamilton Rating Scale for Depression (HRSD)	A significantly greater decrease in depression scores in IPT group
Klier et al., 2001	IPT group setting	Austria	N = 17	Open trial pilot	DSM-IV HRSD EPDS	A significant decrease from baseline to posttreatment for EPDS and HRSD scores

EG = experimental group
CG = control group

(Chen, Tseng, Chou, & Wang, 2000). The primary aim was similar to other support groups described earlier in the chapter, that is, to bring depressed mothers together to share problems and solutions.

Two postpartum depression support groups reported in the literature also included the women's partners. In Australia, a support group program for postpartum depressed mothers and their partners ran for eight sessions for 2 hours each (Morgan et al., 1997). One of the eight sessions focused on the couple. The group sessions for the mothers were led by a female occupational therapist and a nurse, whereas the couples session was also led by these same clinicians plus a male clinical psychologist. Cognitive–behavioral and psychotherapeutic strategies were used to help the couples with their concerns. For the women, their sessions focused on myths of motherhood, postpartum depression, relationships, and mother–infant attachment.

In Canada, the impact of partner support in the treatment of women's postpartum depression was assessed (Misri, Kostaras, Fox, & Kostaras, 2000). Individual support, not group support, was the focus. Postpartum depressed women were seen by a psychiatrist for seven psychoeducational visits. Partners attended visits 2 and 4, where positive interaction between the couple was encouraged. Issues particular to the postpartum period, such as caring for the baby, were the focus.

A 10-week group treatment program in Australia targeting postpartum depression was pilot tested (Meager & Milgrom, 1996). The group treatment contained a combination of social support, educational, and cognitive behavioral components. Each session lasted 1.5 hours and was led by a clinical psychologist. The goals of the program were (1) to decrease postpartum depression and anxiety, (2) to increase mothers self-esteem and help them better adjust to motherhood, (3) to decrease their social and emotional isolation, and (4) to improve their relationships with their partners. One of the sessions involved the spouse so that he could better understand this postpartum mood disorder. After each session, the women were given practical homework assignments to help reinforce the group work.

Secondary Prevention Strategies: Health Visitor Programs

The next category of secondary prevention interventions includes those provided by health visitors, not including support groups already addressed. In the United Kingdom, Cullinan (1991) described a health visitor intervention for women suffering from postpartum depression. Health visitors made six to eight weekly counseling visits. In their listening visits, health visitors listened to postpartum depressed mothers describe their feelings using a nondirective listening approach.

Seeley, Murray, and Cooper (1996) designed and tested a health visitor intervention in both detecting and managing postpartum depression. Health visitors were trained to detect this mood disorder using the EPDS and to treat this mood disorder.

In Sweden, postpartum depressed mothers received six weekly counseling visits by child health clinic nurses (Wickberg & Hwang, 1996). The nurses used nondirective counseling methods and were encouraged to listen instead of giving advice.

Secondary Prevention Strategies: Interpersonal Psychotherapy

IPT was the third category of secondary prevention interventions noted in the literature. Stuart and O'Hara (1995) described IPT for postpartum depression. IPT is based on the belief that mothers who experience social disruptions are at an increased risk for developing postpartum depression. IPT focuses on mothers' interpersonal relationships as the basis for intervention. IPT helps women in changing their relationships or their expectations of those relationships. As Stuart and O'Hara proposed, IPT treats postpartum depressed women on four differing interpersonal problem areas: role transitions, interpersonal disputes, grief, and interpersonal deficits. After an initial assessment, the postpartum depressed mother and the therapist decide on a particular problem area and start addressing it. IPT is a short-term therapy; thus, it is not possible to cover an unlimited number of problematic issues.

In 2000, O'Hara, Stuart, Gorman, and Wenzel assessed the efficacy of IPT for postpartum depression. Postpartum depressed mothers received 12 weeks of IPT, with each session lasting 1 hour. Common problematic areas focused on in IPT were conflicts with partners or their family members, a loss of work relationship and/or social relationships, and other losses related with birth.

IPT has been adapted for the group settling in the treatment of postpartum depression (Klier, Muzik, Rosenblum, & Lenz, 2001). Stages of the postpartum group IPT approach included the following: (1) Initial sessions (numbers 1 and 2) were held with the individual woman to discuss her symptoms and diagnosis of postpartum depression. (2) In middle sessions (numbers 3–9), each individual mother's problem areas were addressed within the group context. Particular intervention strategies are identified. (3) Final sessions (numbers 10–12) focus on the evaluation of the treatment goals and mothers' newly acquired skills.

Secondary Prevention Strategies: Massage and Relaxation Therapy

Massage and relaxation therapy is the last secondary prevention strategy to be described. Field, Grizzle, Scafidi, Abrams, Kuhn, and Schanberg (1996) examined the effects of 10 sessions of massage therapy or relaxation therapy over 5 weeks with adolescents suffering from postpartum depression. Each session lasted for 30 minutes per day on 2 consecutive days per week.

Psychopharmacologic Treatments

As we know, the postpartum period is a time of major hormonal shifts as well as psychologic demands. A strong message from the brain of dysregulation is given if a woman comes to your office complaining of significant symptoms of depression that are getting in the way of her functional living. The priority in her care then is to quiet the brain and treat the dysregulation. Although talk therapy is a major adjunct to physiologic healing, it is my belief (Jeanne) that medication is necessary to help the woman's brain reset and reregulate so that she can get on with the psychosocial and developmental work of becoming a mother. As you have read, significant negative outcomes exist for not only the woman but also for the infant and the family dynamics if this disorder is not treated.

In a critical review of biological interventions for the treatment of postpartum depression, Dennis and Stewart (2004) reported that although tricyclic antidepressants, selective serotonergic reuptake inhibitors (SSRIs), and other antidepressants have been shown to be effective in randomized controlled studies for the treatment of depression in men and women of childbearing age, there is a lack of good studies among postpartum women. Dennis and Stewart reported that there were only four studies that showed that antidepressant medications, especially the SSRIs, may have a therapeutic effect on severely depressed postpartum women (Appleby, Warner, Whitton, & Faragher, 1997; Cohen, Viguera, Bouffard, & Al, 2001; Dennis & Steward, 2004; Suri, Burt, Altshuler, Zuckerbrow-Miller, & Fairbanks, 2001). The recommendation for the use of antidepressant medications in the treatment of postpartum depression is based on the general depression data (Altshuler et al., 2002; Gold, 2002; Hendrick & Gitlin, 2004; Marcus, Barry, Flynn, Tandon, R., & Greden, 2001; Nonacs & Cohen, 1998; Wisner, Parry, & Piontek, 2002).

Based on the expert consensus guidelines published in 2002 (Altshuler et al., 2002), the recommendation for the treatment of the acute phase of a nonpsychotic postpartum depression is the combination of antidepressant medications and psychosocial interventions, whether the mother is breastfeeding or not. They recommend for women with a milder major depression that the treatment with medications and psychosocial support is supported only if the mother is not breastfeeding. There was no first-line consensus on the situation of breastfeeding with milder depression. The combination of antidepressants plus antipsychotic medications was recommended by 94% of the experts for mothers who were not breastfeeding and by 79% for breastfeeding mothers.

In this expert consensus report, the panel suggested, based on data pertaining to lactating women only, that sertraline was the treatment of choice, rated by 97% of the experts, and paroxetine was the other first-line alternative (83%). Tricyclics and fluoxetine were second-line choices but were still rated first line by approximately two thirds of the experts. Half of the experts felt that it was appropriate to measure infant blood levels of antidepressants. The data pertinent to the use of SSRI agents and breastfeeding continue to evolve, and it is the responsibility of the prescribing clinician to be up-to-date on that latest research. A main source of information is the Massachusetts General Hospital Center for Women's Mental Health (www.womensmentalhealth.org) and the Motherisk Program in Toronto, Canada (www.motherisk.org). We have included a chart in the appendix pertaining to medications and breastfeeding. Again, we cannot stress enough that this information is constantly changing and evolving; thus, be sure to secure the current references so that you are up-to-date in your clinical practice. It is also important that if you are referring a woman to a psychopharmacologist that that person be up-to-date on the issues pertaining to postpartum, lactation, and medications.

Electroconvulsant therapy (ECT) was recommended for psychotic depression whether the woman was breastfeeding or not. If the breastfeeding woman had failed to respond to tricyclics, SSRIs, or antipsychotics but had responded to other medications for which there were significant safety concerns (e.g., monoamine oxidase inhibitors (MAOIs)), then the experts strongly recommended the use of ECT (Altshuler et al., 2001).

According to the review by Dennis and Stewart (2004), estrogen therapy has been advocated with preliminary results from two studies (Ahokas, Kaukoranta, & Aito, 1999; Ahokas, Kaukoranta, Wahlbeck, & Aito, 2001; Gregoire, Kumar, Everitt, Henderson, & Studd, 1996). Until better controlled studies are conducted, it is unclear regarding the use of estrogen supplements in the treatment of postpartum depression. The effects of estrogen and breastfeeding women need to be examined, and further research is needed in the aspects of the sex–steroid implications to the etiology of postpartum depression.

Some beginning studies use sleep deprivation as a treatment that may benefit women with postpartum depression (Liebenluft, Moul, Schwartz, Madden, & Wehr, 1993; Parry, Curran, Stuenkel, Yokimozo, Tam, Powell, & Gillin, 2000; Wu & Bunney, 1990). Critically timed sleep deprivation interventions may benefit women with postpartum depression. Currently, the mechanism for the therapeutic effects of sleep deprivation or the differential benefit of late versus early night sleep deprivation is unknown (Dennis & Stewart, 2004). Further research is warranted to explore this potential therapy for women who are experiencing postpartum depression.

Let us go through a case and begin to get a clearer sense of the process of the entire care plan of a woman who enters your practice with symptoms of postpartum depression (major depressive disorder with a postpartum onset).

Case Study

Lorraine calls your office and leaves a message telling you that she had a baby 5 weeks ago and that she is not feeling very well. Her doctor told her to call you because he thinks she has postpartum depression. She asks that you call her back and answer some questions that she is having regarding how she feels. You return the call and ask Lorraine how you can help her. She is very quiet on the phone, and at times she seems to be breathing deeper and sighing. You know that a critical aspect of this first contact with this woman will influence the progress of this interaction. Your goal is to establish rapport and empathic connection. You ask Lorraine to share with you what has been going on and how you can help her.

Lorraine begins by telling you that she had a baby 5 weeks ago and that she does not know what is going on. "I really wanted to be a mother and now I don't know if this was such a good idea. I don't feel very well. I feel like I am jumping out of my skin. I can't settle down. I pace around most of the time. I don't really feel any connection to the baby. I mean that I take care of him, but there doesn't seem to be any love. . . . All I want to do is sleep, and I am scared. I have never felt like this." You are listening to her, and you know that the fact that she called is critical and that you need to support her feelings and to remember that it is her reality. Do not move in with problem-solving strategies too quickly.

You know that you need to see Lorraine in your office. Let her know that in your opinion it sounds like she is having a difficult time and that you would be happy to see her. You then move to a bit of normalization by sharing with her that many women experience difficulties after they give birth but that, unfortunately, we do not talk very much about it. It seems that everyone does well after birth. She deserves to feel well, and you are very glad that she called. Can she come to your office tomorrow with her baby and partner for a total evaluation?

She arrives the next day, and you greet her and bring her into your office. Lorraine brought her 5-week-old son and her partner, Tim. They sit across from you, and you see that they look exhausted and a bit scared. Lorraine does not maintain eye contact, and Tim begins the conversation. "I don't know what is going on. Lorraine is having such a difficult time, and she is such a strong woman. What is going on? We really wanted this baby, and now I am not sure that was such a good idea. I am really worried about her."

You look at Lorraine and Tim and share with them that you are going to be asking a significant amount of questions to find out what is going on and how you can help. You know that they are having a difficult time, and you are glad that they called you. The assessment process begins by collecting the current data and then the history. My approach is to try to understand what has been happening through her life to cause the vulnerability that has resulted in some dysregulation in her biology at this time, in addition to the normal biological changes of pregnancy and postpartum. What is the level of brain strain (Sichel & Driscoll, 1999) that she is experiencing?

Lorraine describes that she is 32 years old and that she and Tim have been together for 5 years. She was working full time as a nurse up to the day of delivery, and she had an unremarkable pregnancy. She got pregnant after 3 months of trying. The couple attended childbirth classes. The birth was exciting, and they were thrilled. "I don't know what happened then. I was feeling so happy. I was tired, but I felt connected and happy to have a son. He is so cute. Now I am feeling disconnected, not very happy, and I am not so sure this was such a good plan."

I again told Lorraine that I was going to ask her a lot of questions, and I explained that my rationale was to find out how her brain got to this point. It is was my belief that there are multiple factors that lead to postpartum depression and that we had to find out how this pregnancy and postpartum affected her brain biochemistry, and in essence try to learn how her life had led her to my office. I explained the earthquake assessment model and that I would be collecting data on the three domains: reproductive hormones, stress hormones, and family history. We began. I asked her whether she wanted Tim to stay or go outside, as we could call him back after we collected the information. "No, he can stay. I don't have any secrets from Tim." I also shared with her that I had been a lactation consultant in the past and that she could nurse the baby in my presence when he was hungry if she desired. I could also try to answer any questions that she had regarding lactation and breastfeeding.

We began the assessment with a genetic (family) history. I find that this area is sometimes easier to talk about. Lorraine stated that her 65-year-old father was alive and had just retired from his job as a policeman. He was currently being treated for atrial fibrillation but had no significant medical history, and Lorraine described that he had no history of mental illness. She described him as steady, available, and close to her. She felt that her parents had a nice marriage and seemed to like each other. Her mother did have a history of mood and anxiety disorders that occurred when she was going through the change. Her mother was currently 62 years old and experienced severe anxiety when she was perimenopausal. She was treated with sertraline, which helped her a lot. Lorraine had never asked her about her postpartum experiences in depth but said that she would do so now that we were talking about it.

She did not know of any mental illness in the extended family and verbalized that the family was connected and that everyone seemed to like each other. Then it was time to ask her about her history—what her life was like so that we could develop the longitudinal assessment. I wanted to hear her story.

Lorraine sat up straight and seemed very engaged in this process. I asked her what she could remember from the early days of her life (0 to 5 years of age). She denied any significant history that she could remember. She did have a sister who was born when she was 3 years old but did not remember any problems with that. "My sister and I are very close." When we moved into school age, she recalled that they had moved when she was in the fourth grade and had to go to a different school. "I hated that. I had left all my friends and did not know anyone; luckily, my sister was going to the same school, so we helped each other. I do not remember how long it took me to adjust, but then I stayed in that school until 8th grade." Next was her memory of any significant events in high school: relationships, school experiences, alcohol, drug use, etc. Lorraine described an event with a boyfriend. They had been dating for a while. He was a bit "possessive," and they would have little fights about that all the time. "One time he was so mad that he tried to choke me. I was terrified, and in reality, so was he. We took a timeout after that, and I really did not want to go out with him anymore. We did continue for a while, but I was always a bit anxious around him. Ultimately, we broke up, and that was okay. He didn't bother me anymore." She graduated from high school and was accepted to a nursing school out of state. "I was both excited and terrified of that, as I had never been away from home before."

Nursing school was described as an ultimately good experience, but she described severe homesickness during the first semester. She was anxious and sad. "I would call my parents a lot just to talk to them. I would cry and kept wondering whether it was such a good idea to go away to school. Finally, I met a really nice girl who was also a bit shy and anxious, and we began to hang around together. Gradually, we both began to feel better. In fact, she was my roommate for my entire school experience, and we are still best friends. She had a baby last year and has been very supportive. She kept telling me to call the doctor because of how I felt. "Why is this happening to me? I didn't ask for this. I just wanted to have a baby, become a family, and have a nice time. It doesn't make sense. What did I do to get this?"

She met Tim her senior year in nursing school and then dated for 2 years before they got engaged and married 5 years ago. He is a firefighter. "He is my best friend. I feel so fortunate to have him in my life, but this is scaring him. He doesn't know what to do, nor do I."

We moved into her reproductive history, and I asked Lorraine to describe for me when she got her first period and what the experience was like before she had her first bleeding. She described that she got her first period when she was 15, and she remembered that for a few months before she would get headaches. "It felt like migraines at that time." She would have some stomach aches. When her period did start she would have some uncomfortable symptoms before her menses. "It felt like PMS. I would get irritated, very tired, and easily agitated and wanted to eat a whole bag of potato chips. After my period began, I would feel fine. I just learned to live with that. I tried to eat well, drink lots of water, and decrease my caffeine intake."

I asked Lorraine whether she ever had taken birth control pills. She replied, "Yes, that was a disaster. I took them for 4 months, and those 4 months were the worst. I felt so agitated and sad. It was like the world was waiting for me to pick a fight. I gained weight and just hated them. After 4 months I just stopped them and figured I would have to use condoms and foam as contraceptives, not condoms and the pill. When I stopped them I felt better soon after and just thought that I would not take them again." I was beginning to uncover an extreme sensitivity to hormonal changes with her brain biology. She did not connect the relationship, but I was beginning to hear that connection. When I asked her about her pregnancy, she described that they had decided that they wanted to start a family. Tim was doing well at work, and she was happy in nursing but ready to take some time off and start a family. "I knew I could work after the baby if I wanted to. They always need help at the hospital." The pregnancy was planned, and it took 3 months before she became pregnant. I asked Lorraine to describe the first trimester. "Well, I knew I was pregnant within 2 weeks after missing my last period. I did a home pregnancy test. I was thrilled, and so was Tim. I didn't see my doctor until I was about 11- or 12-weeks pregnant. That trimester was horrific. I was tired and nauseous all of the time, especially in the evening. I would live on crackers and water. I was irritable and really not a very nice person. When I saw the doctor, he just said that it was almost over and that I was going into my second trimester. Things would quiet down then. Well, in my second trimester, I was a nervous wreck. I was trying so hard to relax. I didn't use caffeine. I walked a lot. I tried to rest. I wrote in my journal. I just wasn't sure what was going on. You know, I am a nurse. I should know about this, but it was just strange. In the last trimester, we took childbirth classes, and that made me a bit more anxious. I was worried that I could die. Now, who are you going to tell that to? I didn't even tell Tim that. He would have thought I was nuts. So in some ways, my anxiety shifted. It was focused on the birth, and that seemed to be normal. I was a bit irritable, but again, I blamed it on the pregnancy. I had had feelings like that before, but I never connected them with anything."

I asked her to describe the birth. "I was 39 weeks, and my membranes ruptured in the evening. I had just seen the doctor that day, and he said that the head was down and that everything looked fine. When my membranes ruptured, I called him, and he told me to just stay home and call again when the contractions were about 5 minutes apart. Tim and I were excited, and we made sure that my suitcase and his bag, as he was going to stay with me in the hospital, were ready. We called our families and put them on alert, and we were set to go. By midnight, nothing had happened, so we decided to go to bed. I was to see the doctor in the morning anyway. Well, at 3:00 a.m., I woke up with the biggest contraction. It scared the hell out of me. It was unbelievable, and then the contractions were coming regularly and getting stronger. We were doing our breathing, but I was scared. We called the doctor, and he said that he would meet us at the hospital." She went on to describe the ride to the hospital, the admission procedure, and then the labor and delivery experience. "I was 8 cm when I was admitted. Things were moving quickly. I had thought I might get an epidural, but now it was too late. I was too dilated. Tim was great. He kept trying to help me focus, and the nurse, Sheila, was fantastic. She really helped us focus and maintain some form of control. The pains were intense. Then it was time to push. I did that for an hour, and then he was born. I couldn't believe it. He looked purple and skinny. He weighed 7 pounds 5 ounces and was 20 inches long. Tim was crying, and I was sobbing. I couldn't believe it. He was alive. He had all of his toes and fingers, one nose, two eyes. He was alive, and so was I. I didn't die!"

I asked her to describe her memory of that first day after baby Timmy was born. "Jeanne, I just kept looking at him. He was so perfect. I was amazed at the process. I was still alive, and so was he. All of my worries and fears were for naught. I was exhausted but thrilled. Then we had to make the decision about circumcision. Although Tim and I had discussed this and we both agreed that we wanted it done, I was terrified, and my anxiety came back about that issue. I was able to care for Timmy and felt very comfortable then. Now I am a mess. The breastfeeding went relatively well. I had soreness, but he seemed to get the hang of it as the days went on. I was really engorged when we got home on day 2, but I knew that was normal. Some great nurses helped me and gave me some tips to help get him on with the engorgement. The breastfeeding is fine. It has worked out really well. I love to feed him, but then I look at him and wonder how he is going to grow with a mother who is so anxious and so doubtful. I am scared now. I worry that I might drop him, but more than that, I just feel like I am not a good mother. I am exhausted. I feel like a robot going about the work of caring for a baby—but no connection. The joy and excitement are gone. I think that Tim and Timmy would be better off without me. I am not a good mother, nor am I a good wife." With this, Tim looked at her quickly and said, "What do you mean when you say, 'We would be better off without you?' Lorraine, what do you mean? Do you think of leaving?" Lorraine started to sob at this point. It was like she let go of the biggest burden that she had been carrying. She had broken and told the main secret. She now spoke about guilt and shame for her feelings and how scary it had been to think these things and not be able to talk about them.

I shared with Lorraine that other women experience her feelings, that I felt honored that she was able to share them with Tim and me, and that we would help her feel better. I was able to see that Lorraine had a history of sensitivity to hormonal shifts, had a negative experience to exogenous hormones, and that the pregnancy had really tipped her biochemistry over the edge (see Figure 5.3). Now began the education process to inform them what I felt was going on and how we would treat it. I needed some other basic information: How was she sleeping? She replied that she really does not sleep. She just lies down, waits for the baby to wake, and dozes in and out. She had some diarrhea, has been having headaches for the past few weeks, and is taking acetaminophen regularly. She has been having Diet Cokes, thinking that the caffeine will help her to get more focused.

I shared with Lorraine and Tim that I thought she had a depression with anxiety and that we would need to collaborate on a care plan that would help her to manage her symptoms and feel better. I shared with her the Earthquake Assessment and explained McEwen's concept of Allostatic Loading, how that impacts our brain, and that the brain will then emit

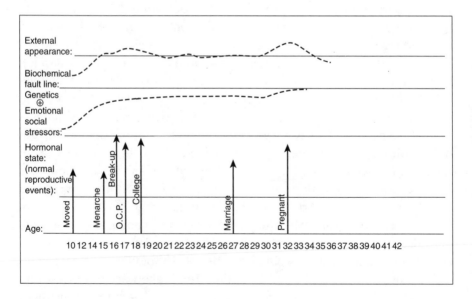

Figure 5.3 The Earthquake Assessment: Lorraine
Sichel, D. & Driscoll, J. S.: *Women's Moods: What every woman must know about hormones, the brain, and emotional health.* 1999. By permission of HarperCollins Publishers, Inc., p. 100.

symptoms to tell us that it is not doing that well. I explained that the treatment usually involved helping her get to sleep, the use of antidepressants, and therapy. My opinion was that she needed both to help her brain get reregulated so that she could go on with the work of becoming a mother. We would use the therapy as a place for her to share her feelings. She was told that she was safe to say whatever she was feeling. We would also talk about adjustment to motherhood and how postpartum is an experience of role change and role transition that involves sadness as we say goodbye to who we were and say hello to who we are becoming. I shared with her that I would want her to come weekly for a while. Then we could reevaluate the frequency when she felt better. She was told that she could call me with any questions and that nothing was unintelligent. We began to develop her NURSE Program (Sichel & Driscoll, 1999).

NURSE Program

- **N**ourishment and needs: We went over Lorraine's diet to ascertain her daily intake of protein, fruits, vegetables, and carbohydrates. We discussed the need to increase her protein intake and gave suggestions of how to aim for short, frequent feedings (yogurt, rolled turkey, roast beef, and fruit).
  - Fluid intake: wean from caffeine, increase water intake to 8 to 10 ounce glasses of water per day
  - Vitamins: continue prenatals if she still had any and then take a daily multivitamin, omega 3-fatty acids, vitamin E (400 IU), and vitamin C (500 mg)
  - Medications:
    - Benzodiazepines: I was going to prescribe a very small dose of Clonazepam (Klonopin)(0.5 mg) for her to take at bedtime, with the hope that she would get into a deep sleep. We discussed the use of pumped breast milk or formula depending on her informed choice.
    - Antidepressants: I was going to prescribe an SSRI to help with the anxiety and depression, and we discussed the choices in relationship to her breastfeeding experience. We would start on a very low starting dose and increase gently over time. The other issue is that these medications do not work quickly. It takes

about 4 to 8 weeks to achieve therapeutic benefit, but we would be working together to support that with other strategies in collaboration. (I use cognitive strategies, restructuring techniques, and group support.)

- **U**nderstanding: We discussed the multiple factors that can lead to postpartum depression, and I shared with her the trajectory of healing that I had observed from my patients over the years. There were books that she could read as well as web sites (Summers & Logsdon, 2005) that could be accessed via her computer at a later date, but I felt that we did not want to overwhelm her with too much information at this time. She needed to know that any question was important and that I was going to be with her through this healing process.
  - ○ Journal keeping was encouraged.
  - ○ Weekly therapy sessions were begun.

- **R**est and relaxation: We discussed the need for restorative sleep and how the Clonazepam would be useful in the beginning. Eventually, however, the SSRI would help to quiet her brain, and her sleep should be better over time. We discussed strategies of resting in the day and securing help from relatives and friends to watch the baby so that she could rest and allow her brain to go "off call."
- **S**pirituality: I ascertained that Lorraine had a strong belief in God, although she was not practicing in any organized religion. She found that prayer was very helpful to her, and I encouraged her to continue what she felt supported her.
- **E**xercise: Lorraine had exercised regularly before the pregnancy and the birth. We discussed walks that she could take around her neighborhood, both with the baby in the carriage and without. It was important for her to get outside and move her body, as exercise can increase the secretion of endorphins in the brain, and those hormones help people feel better.

We agreed to meet next week. I ended by asking whether either of them had any questions. I told them that they could call me with any concerns, questions, and/or worries. When I saw Lorraine a week later, she had slept for at least 5 hours consecutively at night but was not feeling significantly better with regard to her connection, or rather lack of connection, with Timmy. She still described self-disparaging thoughts and negative self-talk. We increased her SSRI each week, and by the sixth week, Lorraine was describing times when she was laughing and felt light hearted. "But then I would get anxious and couldn't believe that it would last. I was waiting for the darkness to descend again." We discussed the healing trajectory and the process that it involves.

References

Affonso, D. D., De, A. K., Horowitz, J. A., & Mayberry, L. J. (2000). An international study exploring levels of postpartum depressive symptomatology. *Journal of Psychosomatic Research, 49,* 207–216.

Achenbach, T. M. (1991). *Manual for the Child Behavior Checklist 4-18 and 1991 Profile.* Burlington: University of Vermont Department of Psychiatry.

Ahokas, A., Kaukoranta, J., & Aito, M. (1999). Effect of oestradiol on postpartum depression. *Psychopharmacology* (Berl), 146, 108–110.

Ahokas, A., Kaukoranta, J., Wahlbeck, K., & Aito, M.. (2001). Estrogen deficiency in severe postpartum depression: Successful treatment with sublingual physiologic 17b-estradiol: A preliminary study. *Journal of Clinical Psychiatry,* 62, 332–336.

Altshuler, L., Cohen, L. S., Moline, M. L., Kahn, D. A., Carpenter, D., Docherty, J. P. & Ross, R.W. (2002). Expert consensus guidelines for the treatment of depression in women: A new treatment tool. *MentalFitness,* 1, 69-83.

Amankwaa, L. C. (2003). Postpartum depression among African-American women. *Issues in Mental Health Nursing,* 24, 297–316.

American Psychiatric Association (2000). *Diagnostic and statistical manual of mental disorders.* (4th ed.). Text revision. Washington, DC: author.

Appleby, L., Warner, R., Whitton, A., & Faragher, B. (1997). A controlled study of fluoxetine and cognitive-behavioral counseling in the treatment of postnatal depression. *British Medical Journal,* 314, 932–936.

Areias, M. E., Kumar, R., Barros, N., & Figueiredo, E. (1996). Correlates of postnatal depression in mothers and fathers. *British Journal of Psychiatry,* 169, 36–41.

Barnet, B., Joffe, A., Duggan, A. K., Wilson, M. D., & Repke, J. T. (1996). Depressive symptoms, stress, and social support in pregnant and postpartum adolescents. *Archives of Pediatric and Adolescent Medicine,* 150, 64–69.

Bayley, N. (1969). *The Bayley Scales on infant development.* New York: Psychological Corporation.

Beck, C.T. (1993). Teetering on the Edge: A substantive theory of postpartum depression. *Nursing Research,* 42, 42-48.

Beck, C. T. (1995). The effects of postpartum depression on maternal-infant interaction: A meta-analysis. *Nursing Research,* 44, 298–304.

Beck, C. T. (1996a). A meta-analysis of predictors of postpartum depression. *Nursing Research,* 45, 297–303.

Beck, C. T. (1996b). A meta-analysis of the relationship between postpartum depression and infant temperament. *Nursing Research*, 45, 225–230.

Beck, C. T. (1996c). Postpartum depressed mothers' experiences interacting with their children. *Nursing Research*, 45, 98–104.

Beck, C. T. (1998). The effects of postpartum depression on child development: A meta-analysis. *Archives of Psychiatric Nursing*, 12, 12–20.

Beck, C. T. (2001). Predictors of postpartum depression: An update. *Nursing Research*, 50, 275–285.

Beck, C. T. (2002). Postpartum depression: A metasynthesis. *Qualitative Health Research*, 12, 453–472.

Beck, C. T. (2002). Releasing the pause button: Mothering twins during the first year of life. *Qualitative Health Research*, 12, 593–608.

Beck, C. T. & Gable, R. K. (2002). *Postpartum Depression Screening Scale Manual.* Los Angeles: Western Psychological Services.

Beck, C. T., & Gable, R. K. (2005). Screening performance of the postpartum depression screening scale-Spanish version. *Journal of Transcultural Nursing*, 16.

Beeghly, M., Weinberg, M. K., Loson, K. L., Kernan, H., Riley, J. M., & Tronick, E. Z. (2002). Stability and change in level of maternal depressive symptomatology during the first postpartum year. *Journal of Affective Disorders*, 71, 169–180.

Bhugra, D., & Gregorie, A. (1993). Social factors in the genesis and management of postnatal psychiatric disorders. In D. Bhugra & J. Leff (Eds.), *Principles of social psychiatry.* Oxford: Blackwell.

Boath, E. H., Pryce, A. J., & Cox, J. L. (1998). Postnatal depression: The impact on the family. *Journal of Reproductive and Infant Psychology*, 16, 199–203.

Bond, J. (1995). Post adoption depression syndrome. *Roots and Wings Magazine.* Retrieved from www.adopting.org/pad.html.

Boyce, P. M. (2003). Risk factors for postnatal depression: A review and risk factors in Australian populations. *Archives of Women's Mental Health*, 6, s43–s50.

Bugdayci, R., Sasmaz, C. T., Tezcan, H., Kurt, A. O., & Oner, S. (2004). A cross-sectional prevalence study of depression at various times after delivery in Mersin province in Turkey. *Journal of Women's Health*, 13, 63–68.

Campbell, S. B., & Cohn, J. F. (1997). The timing and chronicity of postpartum depression: Implications for infant development. In P. J. (Ed.), *Postpartum depression and child development* (pp. 165–197). New York: Guilford.

Carpiniello, B., Pariante, C. M., Serri, F., Costa, G., & Carta, M. G. (1997). Validation of the Edinburgh Postnatal Depression Scale in Italy. *Journal of Psychosomatic Obstetric and Gynecology*, 18, 280–285.

Chaaya, M., Campbell, O. M. R., Kak, F. E., Shaar, D., Harb, H., & Kaddour. (2002). Postpartum depression: Prevalence and determinants in Lebanon. *Archives of Women's Mental Health*, 5, 65–72.

Chan, S. W., Levy, V., Chung, T. K. H., & Lee, D. (2002). A qualitative study of the experiences of a group of Hong Kong Chinese women diagnosed with postnatal depression. *Journal of Advanced Nursing*, 39, 571–579.

Chandran, M., Thoryan, P., Muliyil, J., & Abraham, S. (2002). Postpartum depression in a cohort of women from a rural area of Tamil Nadu, India. *British Journal of Psychiatry*, 181, 499–504.

Chen, C. H., Tseng, Y. F., Chou, F. H., & Wang, S. Y. (2000). Effects of support group intervention in postnatally distressed women: A controlled study in Taiwan. *Journal of Psychosomatic Research*, 49, 395–399.

Clemmens, D. A. (2002). Adolescent mothers' depression after the birth of their babies: Weathering the storm. *Adolescence*, 37, 551–565.

Cohen, J. (1988). *Statistical power analysis for the behavioral sciences*. Hillsdale, NJ: Lawrence Erlbaum.

Cohen, L. S., Viguera, A. C., Bouffard, S. M., & Al, E. (2001). Venlafaxine in the treatment of postpartum depression. *Journal of Clinical Psychiatry*, 62, 592–596.

Cox, J. L. (1979). Amakirs: A Ugandan puerperal psychosis? *Social Psychiatry*, 14, 49–52.

Cox, J. L. (1983). Postnatal depression: A comparison of Scottish and African women. *Social Psychiatry*, 18, 25–28.

Cox, J. L., Holden, J. M., & Sagovsky, R. (1987). Detection of postnatal depression: Development of the 10-item Edinburgh Postnatal Depression Scale. *British Journal of Psychiatry*, 150, 782–786.

Cullinan, R. (1991). Health visitor intervention in postnatal depression. *Health Visitor*, 64, 412–414.

Danaci, A. E., Dinc, G., Deveci, A., Sen, F. S., Icelli, I. (2002). Postnatal depression in Turkey: Epidemiological and cultural aspects. *Social Psychiatry and Psychiatric Epidemiology*, 37, 125–129.

Davis, D. W., Logsdon, M. C., & Birkmer, J. C. (1996). Types of support expected and received by mothers after their infants' discharge from the NICU. *Comprehensive Issues in Pediatric Nursing*, 19, 263–273.

Davis, L., Edwards, H., Mohay, H., & Wollin, J. (2003). The impact of very premature birth on the psychological health of mothers. *Early Human Development*, 73, 61–70.

Deal, L., & Holt, V. (1998). Young maternal age and depressive symptoms: Results from the 1988 National Maternal and Infant Health Survey. *American Journal of Public Health*, 88, 266–270.

Deater-Deckard, K., Pickering, K., Dunn, J. F., & Golding, J. (1998). Family structure and depressive symptoms in men preceding and following the birth of a child: The Avon longitudinal study of pregnancy and childhood study team. *American Journal of Psychiatry*, 153, 818–823.

Dennis, C.-L., E., & Stewart, D. E. (2004). Treatment of postpartum depression, part 1: A critical review of biological interventions. *Journal of Clinical Psychiatry*, 65(9), 1242–1251.

Drewett, R., Blair, P., Emmett, P., Emond, A., & the ALSPAC study team. (2004). Failure to thrive in the term and preterm infants of mothers depressed in the postnatal period: A population-based birth cohort study. *Journal of Child Psychology and Psychiatry*, 45, 359–366.

Driscoll, J. W. (1990). Maternal parenthood and the grief process. *Journal of Perinatal and Neonatal Nursing*, 4, 1–10.

Dudley, M., Roy, K., Kelk, N., & Bernard, D. (2001). Psychological correlatives of depression in fathers and mothers in the first postnatal year. *Journal of Reproductive and Infant Psychology*, 19, 187–202.

Eastwood, P., Horrocks, E., & Jones, K. (1995). Promoting peer group support with postnatally depressed women. *Health Visitor*, 68, 148–150.

Essex, M. J., Klein, M. H., Miech, R., & Smider, N. A. (2001). Timing of initial exposure or maternal major depression and children's mental health symptoms in kindergarten. *British Journal of Psychiatry*, 179, 151–156.

Felice, E., Saliba, J., Grech, V., & Cox, J. (2004). Prevalence rates and psychosocial characteristics associated with depression in pregnancy and postpartum in Maltese women. *Journal of Affective Disorders*, 82, 297–301.

Field, T. (1998). Maternal depression effects on infants and early interventions. *Preventive Medicine*, 27, 200–203.

Field, T., Fox, N., Pickens, J., Nawrocki, T., & Soutullo, D. (1995). Right frontal EEG activation in 3- to 6-month-old infants of "depressed" mothers. *Developmental Psychology*, 31, 358–363.

Field, T., Grizzle, S. F., Abrams, S., & Richardson, M. (1996). Massage therapy for infants of depressed mothers. *Infants Behavior and Development*, 19, 107–112.

Field, T., Grizzle, N., Scafidi, F., Abrams, S., Kuhn, C., & Schanberg, S. (1996). Massage and relaxation therapies' effects on depressed adolescent mothers, *Adolescence*, 31, 903–911.

Fleming, A. S., Klein, E., & Corter, C. (1992). The effects of a social support group on depression, maternal attitudes and behavior in new mothers. *Journal of Child Psychology and Psychiatry*, 33, 685–698.

Foli, K. J., & Thompson, J. R. (2004). *The post-adoption blues*. Emmanus, PA: Rodale, Inc.

Friedman, T., & Gath, D. (1989). The psychiatric consequences of spontaneous abortion. *British Journal of Psychiatry*, 155, 810–813.

Gair, S. (1999). Distress and depression in new motherhood: Research with adoptive mothers highlights important contributing factors. *Child and Family Social Work*, 4, 55–66.

Galler, J. R., Ramsey, F. C., Harrison, R. H., Taylor, J., Cumberbatch, G., & Forde, V. (2004). Postpartum maternal moods and infant size predict performance on a national high school entrance examination. *Journal of Child Psychology and Psychiatry*, 45, 1064–1075.

Garel, M., Blondel, B., Lelong, N., Papin, C., Bonenfant, S., & Kaminski, M. (1992). Depressive reaction after miscarriage. *Contraception, Fertility and Sex*, 20, 75–81.

Gayne, B. N., Gavin, N., Meltzer-Brody, S., Lohr, K. N., Swinson, T., Gartlehner, G., Brody, S., & Miller, W. C. (2005). *Perinatal depression: Prevalence, screening accuracy, and screening outcomes*. Evidence Report/Technology Assessment No.119. (Prepared by RTI-University of North Carolina Evidence-based Practice Center, under Contract No. 290-02-0016). AHRQ Publication No. 05-E006-2. Rockville, MD: Agency for Healthcare Research and Quality.

Gold, L. H. (2002). Postpartum disorders in primary care: Diagnosis and treatment. *Primary Care, 29*, 27–41.

Goodman, J. H. (2004). Postpartum depression beyond the early postpartum period. *Journal of Obstetric, Gynecologic, and Neonatal Nursing, 33*, 410–420.

Goodyer, I. M., Tamplin, A., Herbert, J., & Altham, P. M. (2000). Recent life events, cortisol, dehydroepiandrosterone and the onset of major depression in high-risk adolescents. *British Journal of Psychiatry, 177*, 499–504.

Gregoire, A. J., Kumar, R., Everitt, J., Henderson, A., & Studd, J. (1996). Transdermal oestrogen for treatment of severe postnatal depression. *Lancet, 347*, 918–919.

Halligan, S. L., Herbert, J., Goodyer, I. M., & Murray, L. (2004). Exposure to postnatal depression predicts elevated cortisol in adolescent offspring. *Biological Psychiatry, 55*, 376–381.

Harkness, G. (1995). *Epidemiology in nursing practice.* St. Louis: Mosby.

Harris, T. O., Borsanyi, S., Messari, S., Stanford, K., Brown, G. W., Cleary, S. E., et al. (2000). Morning cortisol as a risk factor for subsequent major depressive disorder in adult women. *British Journal of Psychiatry, 177*, 505–510.

Hay, D. F., Pawlby, S., Angold, A., Harold, G. T., & Sharp, D. (2003). Pathways to violence in the children of mothers who were depressed postpartum. *Developmental Psychology, 39*, 1083–1094.

Heh, S. S., Coombes, L., & Bartlett, H. (2004). The association between depressive symptoms and social support in Taiwanese women during the month. *International Journal of Nursing Studies, 41*, 573–579.

Hendrick, V., & Gitlin, M. J. (2004). *Psychotropic drugs and women: Fast facts.* New York: W. W. Norton & Company.

Hendrick, V., Altshulter, L. L., Strouse, T., & Grosser, S. (2000). Postpartum and nonpostpartum depression: Differences in presentation and response to pharmacologic treatment. *Depression and Anxiety, 11*, 66–72.

Hiscock, H., & Wake, M. (2001). Infant sleep problems and postnatal depression: A community-based study. *Pediatrics, 107*, 1317–1322.

Huang, Y. C., & Mathers, N. (2001). Postnatal depression: Biological or cultural? A comparative study of postnatal women in the UK and Taiwan. *Journal of Advanced Nursing, 33*, 279–287.

Inandi, T., Elci, O. C., Ozturk, A., Egri, M., Polat, A., & Sahin, T. K. (2002). Risk factors for depression in postnatal first year in eastern Turkey. *International Journal of Epidemiology, 31*, 1201–1207.

Jackman, C., McGee, H. M., & Turner, M. (1991). The experience and psychological impact of early miscarriage, *Journal of Psychology, 12*, 108–120.

Janssen, H., Cuisinier, M., Hoogduin, K., & deGraauw, K. (1996). Controlled prospective study on the mental health of women following pregnancy loss. *American Journal of Psychiatry, 153*, 226–230.

Josefsson, A., Berg, G., Nordin, C., & Sydsjo, G. (2001). Prevalence of depressive symptoms in late pregnancy and postpartum. *Acta Obstetrica et Gynecolica Scandinavica, 80*, 251–255.

Kaplan, P. S., Bachorowski, J., Smoski, M. J., & Hudenko, W. J. (2002). Infants of depressed mothers, although competent learners, fail to learn in response to their own mothers' infant-directed speech. *Psychological Science*, 13, 286–271.

Kendell, R. E., Chalmers, J. C., & Platz, C. (1987). Epidemiology of puerperal psychoses. *British Journal of Psychiatry*, 150, 662–673.

Klier, C. M., Muzik, M., Rosenblum, K. L., & Lenz, G. (2001). Interpersonal psychotherapy adapted for the group setting in the treatment of postpartum depression. *Journal of Psychotherapy Practice and Research*, 10, 124–131.

Kumar, R. (1994). Postnatal mental illness: A transcultural perspective. *Social Psychiatry and Psychiatric Epidemiology*, 29, 250–264.

Kumar, C., & Robson, K. M. (1984). A prospective study of emotional disorders in childbearing women. *British Journal of Psychiatry*, 144, 35–47.

Lee, D., Wong, C., Ungvari, G., Cheung, L., Haines, C., & Chung, T. (1997). Screening psychiatric morbidity after miscarriage: Application of the 30-item General Health Questionnaire and the Edinburgh Postnatal Depression Scale. *Psychosomatic Medicine*, 59, 207–210.

Lee, D., Yip, A., Chiu, H., Leung, T., & Chung, T. (2001). A psychiatric epidemiological study of postpartum Chinese women. *American Journal of Psychiatry*, 158, 220–226.

Leonard, L. (1998). Depression and anxiety disorders during multiple pregnancy and parenthood. *Journal of Obstetric, Gynecologic, and Neonatal Nursing*, 27, 329–337.

Liebenluft, E., Moul, D. E., Schwartz, P. J., Madden, P.A., & Wehr, T.A. (1993). A clinical trial of sleep deprivation in combination with antidepressant medication. *Psychiatric Research*, 46, 13–227.

Logsdon, M. (2004). Depression in adolescent girls: Screening and treatment strategies for primary care providers. *Journal of the American Medical Women's Association*, 59, 101–106.

Logsdon, M. C., Davis, D. W., Birkimer, J. C., & Wilkerson, S. A. (1997). Predictors of depression in mothers of preterm infants. *Journal of Social and Behavioral Personality*, 12, 73–88.

Lovestone, S., & Kumar, R. (1993). Postnatal psychiatric illness: The impact on partners. *British Journal of Psychiatry*, 163, 210–216.

Luoma, I., Tamminen, T., Kaukonen, P., Laippala, P., Puura, K., Salmelin, R., & Almqvist, F. (2001). Longitudinal study of maternal depressive symptoms and child well-being. *Journal of American Academy of Child Adolescent Psychiatry*, 40, 1367–1374.

Marcus, S. M., Barry, K. L., Flynn, H. A., Tandon, R., & Greden, J. F. (2001). Treatment guidelines for depression in pregnancy. *International Journal of Gynaecology and Obstetrics*, 72, 61–70.

Matthey, S., Barnett, B., Ungerer, J., & Waters, B. (2000). Paternal and maternal depressed mood during the transition to parenthood. *Journal of Affective Disorders*, 60, 75–85.

Mauthner, N. (1993). Towards a feminist understanding of postnatal depression. *Feminism & Psychology*, 3, 350–355.

McCarthy, D. (1972). *Manual for the McCarthy Scales of Children's Abilities.* New York: Psychological Corporation.

McCarthy, H. (2000). Post-adoption depression: The unacknowledged hazard. Retrieved from http://www.eeadopt.org/home/services/research/pad.survey/.

Meager, I., & Milgram, J. (1996). Group treatment for postpartum depression: A pilot study. *Australian and New Zealand Journal of Psychiatry, 30,* 852–860.

Meignan, M., Davis, M. W., Thomas, S. P., & Droppleman, P. G. (1999). Living with postpartum depression: The father's experience. *MCN: The American Journal of Maternal Child Nursing, 24,* 202–208.

Melges, F. T. (1968). Postpartum psychiatric syndromes. *Psychosomatic Medicine, 30,* 95–108.

Miller, L. (1988). Depression among pregnant adolescents. *Psychiatric Services, 49,* 970.

Misri, S., Kostaras, X., Fox, D., & Kostaras, D. (2000). The impact of partner support in the treatment of postpartum depression. *Canadian Journal of Psychiatry, 45,* 554–558.

Morgan, M., Matthey, S., Barnett, B., & Richardson, C. (1997). A group programme for postnatally distressed women and their partners. *Journal of Advanced Nursing, 26,* 913–920.

Murray, L. (1992). The impact of postnatal depression on infant development. *Journal of Child Psychology and Psychiatry, 33,* 543–561.

Murray, L., & Cooper, P. J. (1997). *Postpartum depression and child development.* New York: The Guilford Press.

Murray, L., Fiori-Cowley, A., Hooper, R., & Cooper, P. (1996a). The impact of postnatal depression and associated adversity on early mother–infant interaction and later infant outcome. *Child Development, 67,* 2512–2526.

Murray, L., Hipwell, A., Hooper, R., Stein, A., & Cooper, P. J. (1996b). The cognitive development of 5-year-old children of postnatally depressed mothers. *Journal of Child Psychology and Psychiatry, 37,* 927–935.

Murray, L., Sinclair, D., Turner, P., Ducournau, P., Stern, A., & Cooper, P. (1999). The socio-emotional development of 5 year old children of postnatally depressed mothers. *Journal of Child Psychology and Psychiatry, 40,* 1259–1272.

Neugebauer, R., Kline, J., O'Connor, P., Shrout, P., Johnson, J., Skodol, A., et al. (1992). Determinants of depressive symptoms in the early weeks after miscarriage, *American Journal of Public Health, 82,* 1332–1339.

Nhiwatiwa, S., Patel, V., & Acuda, W. (1998). Predicting postnatal mental disorder with a screening questionnaire: A prospective cohort study from Zimbabwe. *Journal of Epidemiology and Community Health, 52,* 262–266.

Nonacs, R., & Cohen, L. S. (1998). Postpartum mood disorders: Diagnosis and treatment guidelines. *Journal of Clinical Psychiatry, 59*(Suppl 2), 34–40.

Oates, M. R., Cox, J. L., Neena, S., Asten, P., Glangeud-Freudenthal, N., Figueiredo, B. et al. (2004). Postnatal depression across countries and cultures: A qualitative study. *British Journal of Psychiatry, 184*(Suppl 46), 510–516.

O'Hara, M. W., & Swain, A. M. (1996). Rates and risk of postpartum depression: A meta-analysis. *International Review of Psychiatry, 8,* 37–54.

O'Hara, M. W., Stuart, S., Gorman, L. L., & Wenzel, A. (2000). Efficacy of interpersonal psychotherapy for postpartum depression. *Archives of General Psychiatry, 57,* 1039–1045.

Orozco, E. A. (1995). How *depression interacts with coping resources among African American women.* Unpublished doctoral dissertation, Kent State University, Kent, Ohio.

Parry, B. L., Curran, M. I., Stuenkel, C. A., Yokimozo, M., Tam, L., Powell, K. A., & Gillin, J. C. (2000). Can critically timed sleep deprivation be useful in pregnancy and postpartum depressions? *Journal of Affective Disorders, 60,* 201–212.

Patel, V., Rodrigues, M., & DeSouza, N. (2002). Gender, poverty and postnatal depression: A study of mothers in Goa, India. *American Journal of Psychiatry, 159,* 43–47.

Pickens, J., & Field, T. (1993). Attention getting vs. imitation effects on depressed mother–infant interactions. *Infant Mental Health Journal, 14,* 171–181.

Pillsbury, B. L. K. (1978). "Doing the month": Confinement and convalescence of Chinese women after childbirth. *Social Science and Medicine, 12,* 11–22.

Pitts, F. (1995). Comrades in adversity: The group approach. *Health Visitor, 68,* 144–145.

Prettyman, R. J., Cordle, C. J., & Cook, G. D. (1993). A three-month follow-up of psychological morbidity after early miscarriage. *British Journal of Medical Psychology, 66,* 363–372.

Rahman, A., Iqbal, Z., & Harrington, R. (2003). Life events, social support and depression in childbirth: Perspective from a rural community in the developing world. *Psychological Medicine, 33,* 1161–1167.

Regmi, S., Sligl, W., Carter, D., Grut, W., & Seear, M. (2002). A controlled study of postpartum depression among Nepalese women: Validation of the Edinburgh Postpartum Depression Scale in Kathmandu. *Tropical Medicine and International Health, 7,* 378–382.

Righetti-Veltema, M., Conne-Perreard, E., Bousquet, A., & Manzano, J. (2002). Postpartum depression and mother-infant relationship at 3 months old. *Journal of Affective Disorders, 70,* 291–306.

Righetti-Veltema, M., Bousquet, A., & Manzano, J. (2003). Impact of postpartum depressive symptoms on mother and her 18-month old infant. *European Child & Adolescent Psychiatry, 12,* 75–83.

Robertson, E., Grace, S., Wallington, T., & Stewart, D. (2004). Antenatal risk factors for postpartum depression: A synthesis of recent literature. *General Hospital Psychiatry, 26,* 289–295.

Rodrigues, M., Patel, V., Jaswal, S., & de Souza, N. (2003). Listening to mothers: Qualitative studies on motherhood and depression from Goa, India. *Social Science and Medicine, 57,* 1797–1806.

Saisto, T., Salmela-Aro, K., Nurmi, J. E., & Halmeskaki, E. (2001). Psychosocial predictors of disappointment with delivery and puerperal depression. *Acta Obstetrica Gynecologica Scandinavica, 80,* 39–45.

Sandelowski, M., Docherty, S., & Emden, C. (1997). Qualitative meta-synthesis: Issues and techniques. *Research in Nursing & Health*, 20, 365–371.

Seel, R. M. (1986). Birth rite. *Health Visitor*, 59, 182–184.

Seeley, S., Murray, L., & Cooper, P. J. (1996). The outcome for mothers and babies of health visitor intervention. *Health Visitor*, 69, 135–138.

Sharp, D., Hay, D. F., Pawlby, S., Schmucker, G., Allen, H., & Kumar, R. (1995). The impact of postnatal depression on boys' intellectual development. *Journal of Child Psychology and Psychiatry*, 36, 1315–1336.

Shields-Poe, D., & Pinelli, J. (1997). Variables associated with parental stress in neonatal intensive care units. *Neonatal Network*, 16, 29–37.

Sichel, D., & Driscoll, J. W. (1999). *Women's moods: What every woman must know about hormones, the brain, and emotional health*. New York: William Morrow and Company.

Sinclair, D., & Murray, L. (1998). Effects of postnatal depression on children's adjustment to school: Teachers' reports. *British Journal of Psychiatry*, 172, 58–63.

Small, R., Brown, S., Lumley, J., & Astbury, J. (1994). Missing voices: What women say and do about depression after childbirth. *Journal of Reproductive and Infant Psychology*, 12, 89–103.

Stanley, C., Murray, L., & Stein, A. (2004). The effect of postnatal depression on mother–infant interaction, infant response to the still-face perturbation and performance on an instrumental learning task. *Development and Psychopathology*, 16, 1–18.

Stern, G., & Kruckman, L. (1983). Multi-disciplinary perspectives on postpartum depression: An anthropological critique. *Social Science and Medicine*, 17, 1027–1041.

Strauss, A., & Corbin, J. (1990). *Basics of qualitative research: Grounded theory procedures and techniques*. Newbury Park, Ca: Sage Publications.

Stuart, S., & O'Hara M. W. (1995). Interpersonal psychotherapy for postpartum depression: A treatment program. *Journal of Psychotherapy Practice and Research*, 4, 18–29.

Summers, A.L., & Logsdon, C. (2005). Web sites for postpartum depression. *MCN: American Journal of Maternal Child Nursing*, 30, 88-94.

Suri, R., Burt, B. K., Altshuler, L. L., Zuckerbrow-Miller, J., & Fairbanks, L. (2001). Fluvoxamine for postpartum depression [letter]. *American Journal of Psychiatry*, 158, 1739–1740.

Swanson, K. M. (2000). Predicting depressive symptoms after miscarriage: A path analysis based on the Lazarus paradigm. *Journal of Women's Health & Gender-Based Medicine*, 9, 191–206.

Thapar, A. K., & Thapar, A. (1992). Psychological sequelae of miscarriage: A controlled study using the General Health Questionnaire and the Hospital Anxiety and Depression Scale. *British Journal of General Practice*, 42, 94–96.

Thorpe, K., Golding, J., MacGillivray, I., & Greenwood, R. (1991). Comparison of prevalence of depression in mothers of twins and mothers of singletons. *British Medical Journal*, 302, 875–878.

VanPutten, R., & LaWall, J. (1981). Postpartum psychosis in an adoptive mother and in a father. *Psychosomatics, 22,* 1087–1089.

Veddovi, M., Kerry, D. T., Gibson, F., Bowen, J., & Starte, D. (2001). The relationship between depressive symptoms following premature birth, mothers' coping style, and knowledge of infant development. *Journal of Reproductive and Infant Psychology, 19,* 313–323.

Victoroff, V. (1952). Dynamics and management of parapartum neuropathic reactions. *Diseases of the Nervous System, 13,* 291–298.

White, P. M. (2004). Heat, balance, humors, and ghosts: Postpartum in Cambodia. *Health Care for Women International, 25,* 179–194.

Wickberg, B., & Hwang, C. P. (1996). Counseling of postnatal depression: A controlled study on a population based Swedish sample. *Journal of Affective Disorders, 39,* 209–216.

Victoroff, V. (1952). Dynamics and management of parapartum neuropathic reactions. *Diseases of the Nervous System, 13,* 291–298.

Wisner, K. L., Parry, B. L., & Piontek, C. M. (2002). Postpartum depression. *New England Journal of Medicine, 347,* 194–199.

Wisner, K. L., Perel, J. M., Peindl, K. S., & Hanusa, B. H. (2004). Timing of depressive recurrence in the first year after birth. *Journal of Affective Disorders, 78,* 249–252.

Wolf, A. W., DeAndraca, I., & Lozoff, B. (2002). Maternal depression in three Latin American samples. *Social Psychiatry and Psychiatric Epidemiology, 37,* 169–176.

Wu, J. C., & Bunney, W. E. (1990). The biological basis of an antidepressant response to sleep deprivation and relapse: review and hypothesis. *American Journal of Psychiatry, 147,* 14–21.

Yamashita, H., Yoshida, K., Nakano, H., & Tashiro, N. (2000). Postnatal depression in Japanese women: Detecting the early onset of postnatal depression by closely monitoring the postpartum mood. *Journal of Affective Disorders, 58,* 145–154.

Zelkowitz, P., & Milet, T. H. (2001). The course of postpartum psychiatric disorders in women and their partners. *Journal of Nervous and Mental Disease, 189,* 575–582.

CHAPTER 6

THE POSTPARTUM-DEPRESSION IMPOSTOR: BIPOLAR II DISORDER

Diagnostic Criteria for Bipolar II Disorder

A. Presence (or history) of one or more major depressive episodes.

B. Presence (or history) of at least one hypomanic episode.

C. There has never been a manic episode or a mixed episode.

D. The mood symptoms in criteria A and B are not better accounted for by schizoaffective disorder and are not superimposed on schizophrenia, schizophreniform disorder, delusional disorder, or psychotic disorder not otherwise specified.

E. The symptoms cause clinically significant distress or impairment in social, occupational, or other important areas of functioning. Specify current or most recent episode:

Hypomanic: if currently (or most recently) in a hypomanic episode

Depressed: if currently (or most recently) in a major depressive episode (American Psychiatric Association, 2000, p. 397)

Reprinted with permission from the *Diagnostic and Statistical Manual of Mental Disorders*, Copyright 2000. American Psychiatric Association.

Introduction

In this chapter, bipolar II disorder, the postpartum depression impostor, is discussed. The assessment process and suggested treatment strategies are presented, as well as some of the results from Jeanne's dissertation, *The Experience of Women Living with Bipolar II Disorder*.

Bipolar II disorder is a subtype of bipolar disorder and affects approximately 0.5% of the population and appears to be more common in women (Benazzi, 1999; Mitchell et al., 2001; Simpson et al., 1993). The diagnostic label of bipolar II refers to a clinical situation in which the patient presents with a major depressive episode or a history of a major depressive episode, but when interviewed further, she has a history of hypomanic episodes (Akiskal et al., 2000). A hypomanic episode, described in *The Diagnostic and Statistical Manual of Mental Disorders*-IV-TR (American Psychiatric Association, 2000), is a "distinct period of persistently elevated, expansive, or irritable mood, lasting throughout at least 4 days, that is clearly different from the usual nondepressed mood" (p. 171). Further characteristics of a hypomanic episode include three or more (four if the mood is irritable) of the following symptoms that have persisted and been present to a significant degree: inflated self-esteem or grandiosity, a decreased need for sleep, more talkative than usual or pressure to keep talking, a flight of ideas or a subjective experience that thoughts are racing, distractibility, an increase in goal-directed activity or psychomotor agitation, and/or excessive involvement in pleasurable activities that have a high potential for painful consequences (i.e., buying sprees, sexual indiscretions, or foolish business investments). The patient has no history of a manic episode, which is defined by the DSM-IV-TR as a "distinct period of abnormally and persistently elevated, expansive, or irritable mood, lasting at least one week" (American Psychiatric Association, p. 169). Although a manic episode can cause severe functional impairment, a hypomanic episode does not cause severe alterations in functional living but is noticed by family and friends as a change in behavior that is uncharacteristic to that person.

Akiskal et al. (2000) reported that bipolar II disorder represented the most common phenotype of bipolar disorder, and current data indicate that the nodal duration of hypomanic episodes is 2 days, a much shorter episode then is described in the DSM-IV-TR. The researchers feel that recurrent brief hypomanic episodes, with excitation as short as 1 day, when complicated by major depression, should also be classified as a variant of bipolar II. Women diagnosed with bipolar II disorder have more fluctuating moods than those with bipolar I. Women's brains cope with fluctuating effects and levels of estrogen, progesterone, and testosterone, which may make women with bipolar II disorder more vulnerable to severe depression symptoms during postpartum (Sichel & Driscoll, 1999). They are more unstable and temperamental, which introduces a lot of chaos in their personal and professional lives (Akiskal et al., 2000). The number of women who seek psychiatric care is higher than the number of men. The child-bearing years in a woman's life bring with them the highest incidence of the occurrence of psychiatric illness and hospitalization (Kessler et al., 1994).

In 1999, Sichel and Driscoll (1999) coined the term "postpartum depression impostor" in regard to the bipolar II. The common scenario is that women go from doctor to doctor seeking relief from their symptoms without really responding to any of the treatments prescribed. They appear to present with a serious treatment-resistant depression when in actuality they are living with an undiagnosed bipolar II disorder. Clinically, Sichel and Driscoll (1999) described that new mothers with bipolar II disorder often follow an expected course in the days and weeks of early postpartum. They generally describe a hypomanic phase immediately after the birth of their baby, and this is followed by a severe depression a few weeks later.

As stated previously, bipolar II disorder is a subtype of bipolar disorder and appears to occur more commonly in women. The accurate diagnosis of bipolar II disorder is dependent on the memory of the patient and how the clinician phrases the questions pertaining to the hypomanic episodes. In other words, the experience and skills of the clinician in eliciting the life history and course of the patients' illness have a positive correlation with diagnosis of this disorder. If one considers the elements of a hypomanic episode, it is easy to understand why a woman with a propensity for depressive moods would not seek help from a mental health provider when she experiences a short period of goal-directed energy. She would probably not even view it as a negative experience and, therefore, would never tell anyone. These brief moments are critical to the assessment process and accurate diagnosis of bipolar II disorder. Scrupulous attention must be given to this in the diagnostic process because the choice of a psychotropic agent, if used, depends on the recognition of hypomanic episodes.

Clinicians who were educated to recognize bipolar II far outperformed the structured clinical interviews in the diagnosis of bipolar II disorder (Akiskal, 1996). Bipolar II is a complex diagnosis because many of the patients afflicted with this disorder possess an underlying temperamental dysregulation, as well as features of an atypical depression (Akiskal et al., 2000; Dunner, 1992, 2003; Dunner & Fieve, 1974). The clinician has to identify a pattern of cyclic depressions with distinct hypomanic periods as the core unifying or underlying factor in a patient with co-morbid presentations. Often, the affective aspects of the presentation of the patient with a bipolar II disorder extend beyond the elation and depressive symptoms and include, among others, negative arousal states, panic, irritability, and mood lability (Akiskal, 1996).

In 1998, Angst suggested that a broader definition of hypomania might be justified to ascertain bipolar II disorder and bipolar spectrum disorders. His checklist included symptoms of less sleep, more drive, energy, self-confidence, plans, ideas, more talkative than usual, increased social activities and work motivation, increased physical activities, less shy and inhibited, use of more puns and jokes in conversation, and demonstration of faster thinking. Other symptoms in Angst's (1998) checklist were more laughing; more irritability and impatience; increased consumption of coffee, cigarettes, and/or alcohol; extremely happy mood; overeuphoric; increased sex drive and interest in sex; and overactivity (shopping, business, telephone use, traveling, driving, and visiting). The overall prevalence of brief hypomania in Angst's (1998) sample was relatively high, at 2.8 %; however, using his expanded criteria, a further 11.3% of the population had subdiagnostic hypomanic symptoms. This change leads one to consider using Angst's (1998) checklist over the standard checklist found in the DSM-IV for a more specific diagnosis.

Women with bipolar disorder were at high risk for an exacerbation of an episode at the postpartum time (Kendell, Chalmers, & Platz, 1987; Kessler et al., 1994). Clinically, however, women have shared with me that they are exquisitely sensitive to exogenous hormones and have often felt devalued by health care providers when they were told that their experiences were not supported by research. Sadly, their experiences are not considered as valid. It is difficult enough to be the woman living with the mood disorder, but to have a critical aspect of your biology ignored by the psychiatric health care team and the primary health care team is unconscionable. Studies regarding the effect of medication on women and the impact of their reproductive hormones have to be conducted. At a minimum, the menstrual cycle, as Leibenluft, Fiero, and Rubinow discussed in 1994, needs to be considered as an independent variable in both assessment and research. Clinically, I have learned by listening to women's experiences that there are times in the menstrual cycle that doses of medication need to be increased and then brought back to baseline. My experience supports the notion that the uniqueness of the woman's biology must be considered in the care plans.

Often, women with an undiagnosed bipolar II disorder have lived through the use of multiple antidepressant agents. The medications fail to treat the symptoms and often "poop out." Sometimes higher doses are needed with minimal impact (Benazzi, 2001). Many women have shared that they had been started on antidepressants by their primary care provider and experienced side effects; thus, they just stopped the medication and did not go back to their provider. With the changes in health care delivery systems and the trend of primary care treatment being the entry into the health care system, primary care providers and women's health providers are diagnosing and treating many women for depression. Often these providers are unaware of bipolar II as a hidden diagnosis, an impostor of depressive disorder (Sichel & Driscoll, 1999). In light of this, many women are incorrectly diagnosed and treated for a major depressive disorder rather than a bipolar II disorder. Hypomanic episodes are not being uncovered, which leads to an inaccurate treatment plan with the potential to cause harm.

Psychotherapy provided concurrently with psychopharmacology can address the psychosocial aspects of living with a chronic psychiatric illness. Women need to have a relational connection with a psychiatric care provider who can care for her through her healing trajectory and teach and guide in the aspects of brain care as described by Sichel and Driscoll (1999).

The research regarding women's specific experience with bipolar II is limited but evolving. The embryonic sex-specific, neurobiologic research speaks about the need to differentiate the sexes. The dynamic interaction of the aspects of genetic biology, reproductive biology, and stress biology need to be respected and honored in the area of diagnosis of psychiatric illness (Legato, 2002; Leibenluft, 1999; Sichel & Driscoll, 1999).

Women with undiagnosed bipolar II disorder often present with a severe depressive disorder during their postpartum experiences. Many of these women have had histories of severe, treatment-resistant depression, which caused them to believe that their mood swings were "just who I am." The women describe that their lives before pregnancy were "normal," but after further questioning, they did have short bursts or periods of energy, irritability, anxiety, rage, insomnia, and excitability. These short-lived periods were followed by a "down" time, which they did not necessarily describe as depression. Women would describe this as what they considered "normal." Who, in fact, would consider those small bursts or periods of mood shift to be abnormal? Everyone has had bad days! The need to obtain a detailed history is mandatory in making this diagnosis.

In my doctoral dissertation (Jeanne), a descriptive, qualitative study regarding the experiences of women living with bipolar II disorder was conducted (Driscoll, 2004). The sample consisted of 11 women ranging in age from 24 to 61 years. Using Colaizzi's (1978) methods of qualitative data analysis, four themes emerged: melancholy to mayhem at the flick of a switch; dwelling in the maze: the journey toward diagnosis and treatment; emerging steadiness: regaining control; and cultivating a new self.

Women described that living with bipolar II was "hell and I wouldn't wish it on my worst enemy." The women described the illness as profound depression with sudden, unpredictable episodes or outbursts of emotional energy. These episodes or outburst switch on like a light switch and are often experienced as times of increased anxiety, irritability, rage, agitation, sleep dysregulation, and noisy brains; and some women described feeling directed, goal focused, and able to get things done. The depressive side of the illness was predominant, however, and women described feelings laden with isolation, fatigue, tearfulness, confusion, cognitive fogginess, helplessness, lack of energy, and/or motivation.

Relationships with family and friends were altered, and many of the women felt that they were to blame for the symptoms and described significant feelings of shame that emerged when they assumed that they were "bad and out of control." The hormonal component of the illness was described by the women in the study in that they felt that there was exacerbation of their symptoms during different phases of their menstrual cycle, with the use of oral contraceptives, during perimenopause, and during the menopausal phase of their reproductive lives.

The journey toward diagnosis and treatment was full of obstacles, frustrations, and disappointments. Women described seeing many health care providers and struggling to find providers who would listen to their personal story rather than trying to label them with a diagnosis of depression. They felt misunderstood by providers and often embarked on what one woman described as the "antidepressant shuffle." The women described multiple medication trials (with antidepressant agents) with short-term effects, multiple side effects and feeling caught in a spiral of treatment methods with limited results. The treatment of the illness in many ways mirrored the emotions of the women's experiences: unpredictability, anger, sadness, depression, confusion, and frustration. The paradox was that their feelings in trying to treat the illness were indeed the symptoms that brought them to the providers in the first place.

After the correct medication was found, women described a sense of relief, but the process of trusting the treatment method (mood-stabilizing agents) and regaining control of their lives was lengthy. They had to come to grips with the shame and stigma of the illness and negotiate repair work on relationships with themselves, family, and friends. They voiced extreme concern regarding the impact of their illness on their children as well as the genetic aspects of bipolar II disorder.

The women learned the key aspects of self-care that were mandatory to maintain their health: exercise, healthy diet, adequate sleep, and a connected, empathic health care team. The acceptance of the disorder and the process of living with it was an ongoing process.

Assessment

In order to diagnose bipolar II disorder accurately, a thorough assessment must be made. Attention to the longitudinal history via the Earthquake Assessment (Sichel & Driscoll, 1999) is mandatory to ascertain any hypomanic episodes as well as hormonal exacerbations of symptoms and genetic high-risk factors. Bipolar II disorder poses a particular problem in diagnosis (Bowden, 2001). Bowden feels that the DSM-IV criteria for hypomania are too restrictive in that they require the full symptom picture of mania and duration of symptoms for at least 4 days. The nodal duration of a hypomanic state is 1 to 3 days (Akiskal, 1996). Additionally, many people who seek treatment with bipolar II disorder do so when they are depressed and do not recall any hypomanic episodes or view those episodes as within the range of normal, even desired, function (Bowden, 2001). The consequence of these factors is that many people with bipolar II or similar mild forms of bipolar illness are temporarily or permanently seen as having a unipolar depression, which will consequently lead to the inappropriate use of antidepressants as a psychopharmacologic treatment.

In my dissertation research, many of the women described that the "hypomanic episodes" were times when they felt that they were normal and feeling what "other people feel." One woman said that she felt that it was when she had her "high" that she could get things done—her housework, crafts with her children, and projects. Thus, in her mind, that was a normal mood. She did not consider it a "hypomanic episode." She felt that clinicians need to ask more specific questions about what they describe as high.

It can be useful in the assessment process to ask whether anyone in the woman's family or acquaintances has noticed any symptoms that represent hypomanic symptoms. Some people with bipolar II disorder have mild manic symptoms but have a general hypothymic temperament, which is evidenced by high energy, high capacity for productive work, impatience, and a tendency to get easily annoyed (Bowden, 2001). Family history is essential, as many patients have a family history of bipolarity, although it may not be officially diagnosed. The patient's age is an important factor because a correlation seems to exist between early onsets of symptoms as indicative of bipolar diathesis. Atypical features of depression such as excessive sleeping, overeating, or weight gain can also raise the red flag as a sign of a bipolar sensitivity (Lewis, 2004). Treatment response to antidepressants often delineates the depressive disorders: unipolar and bipolar. A "too good to be true" or a "too soon to be true" response to antidepressants is often an indicator of bipolarity, as the antidepressant medication may cause a treatment-emergent hypomania or mania (Lewis, 2004).

Treatment

The treatment of bipolar II disorder generally includes the use of the mood-stabilizing agents, atypical neuroleptics, benzodiazepines, and occasionally, the augmentation with low doses of antidepressant medication (Hirshfeld et al., 2002). The individuality of the patient must be taken into consideration, and the pharmacologic treatment plan is managed cautiously and closely.

"The uncertainty surrounding the diagnosis of bipolar II extends into decisions about its treatment" (Hadjipavlou, Mok, & Yatham, 2004). Hadjipavlou et al. conducted a systematic review of recent published data regarding the evidence that was published specific to the pharmacotherapy of bipolar II disorder. They reported that there was a lack of good-quality evidence to help clinicians with regard to psychopharmacologic choices and bipolar II. Lamotrigine is the only agent that has demonstrated efficacy in a double-blind randomized clinical trial (RCT), but generalizability was not established (Calabrese, Suppes, Bowden, & Al, 2000). Lithium in long-term therapy, based on observational studies, encouraged the authors of the use of lithium in the treatment of bipolar II disorder (Hadjipavlou et al.). There was some limited support for the use of risperidone in hypomania and for the use of venlafaxine, fluoxetine, and divalproex in treating depression; however, no long-term data exist (Hadjipavlou et al.). The authors commented that the current clinical debate about the use of antidepressants as monotherapy or in combination with a mood stabilizer has yet to be determined. Their final suggestion is that decisions regarding treatment need to be made on a case-by-case basis, individualizing the care of the patient and his or her own unique presentation of the disorder.

As we know, the aim of psychopharmacologic interventions is to treat the neurochemical imbalance of the brain. The major class of drugs that is used in the treatment of bipolar disorders is the mood stabilizers/anticonvulsants.

These include but are not limited to lithium, carbamazepine, valproate, lamotrigine, gabapentin, topiramate (Hirschfeld et al., 2002; Lewis, 2004). Antidepressants may be used, but it is imperative to start the dose low and advance slowly, as there is the potential to induce mania if there is an underlying bipolar diathesis (Amsterdam & Brunswick, 2003; Ghaemi, Hsu, Soldani, & Goodwin, 2003; Goldberger & Truman, 2003; Post et al., 2003). Atypical antipsychotics (olanzapine, risperidone, quetiapine, to name a few) have also been used in the treatment of bipolar II disorders. The psychopharmacologic treatments of bipolar II disorder are based on the individual presentation of symptoms, as there is no specific standard of care.

Breastfeeding with psychopharmacologic agents is a large concern in the care of women with bipolar II disorder because limited data exist about the safety of the mood-stabilizing agents and the neuroleptics on the infant. The data are evolving, and clinicians must be up-to-date on the latest research in this area to provide the information for the woman so that she can make an informed decision about her choice of feeding method (see the appendix on medications and lactation).

Although pharmacotherapy is a major aspect of the treatment plan, other forms of psychotherapy are important components of the treatment plan, as patients with bipolar disorders suffer from psychosocial consequences of their disorder. Psychotherapeutic treatments are aimed at reducing distress and improving their functioning. Some of these include but are not limited to cognitive behavioral therapy, interpersonal therapy, family therapy, psychoeducational strategies, and supportive psychotherapy (Altshuler et al., 2002; Hirschfeld et al., 2002).

Bipolar II disorder is difficult to diagnose, and unless you are considering it as an option, you may be remiss in the data collection that is so important to the identification. Because it is difficult to discern quickly, those who use antidepressant medications and those who may be have a bipolar sensitivity must start the dose very low and increase slowly.

Case Study

Reilly is 34 years old. She is 6 months postpartum and has been complaining of symptoms of depression for some time now. "I just kept hoping that I would feel better. I am trying so hard, but it just seems to be getting harder and harder to hold it together." She has a baby boy, Aden, and had planned to go back to work this month, but "I just can't get my act together. It is so hard to get to sleep. I just keep worrying about everything."

The assessment interview takes about 2 hours using the Earthquake Assessment (Sichel & Driscoll, 1999). Using this model, I collect the pertinent data to how life stressors, family history, and reproductive events have contributed to the state of the woman's brain. We want to know how the woman's brain got here. What is her brain telling us?

Reilly shared with me that 6 months ago she had given birth to her son, Aden. He was "the light of my life," but it was "his birth that seemed to change my whole life." She described that postpartum had been great until about 6 or 7 weeks. "Then I just couldn't function. All I wanted to do was sleep. I cried. Poor Aden—I had no patience for him. My partner thinks I am losing my mind." She called her obstetrician, who prescribed some sertraline for her. "He said that I sounded depressed. I felt better and had more energy but had some side effects of fatigue, nausea, and headaches. We tried another antidepressant. I did feel better again, but then that went away. I got into therapy. I really like my therapist, and she has been so helpful. It is so nice to have a place to talk. We have been working with strategies to get me through the day. Some days I feel as though I am getting better, but then the darkness comes again."

At this point, I noted a few critical pieces of information: Reilly has been on a few antidepressants and had some therapeutic effect but not sustainable. She had a great postpartum for a few weeks. I knew I needed more information about what "great" was, and she also described some days when she felt back to herself. Was she having hypomanic episodes? After a short time of letting her tell me her current story, we came to an appropriate point in the conversation to begin to conduct my assessment interview. I told Reilly that I needed to get a better sense of who she was and what her story was from birth to this phase and stage of her life. We began.

Reilly's parents were both alive and well. Her mother is 63 years old and described by Reilly as "my best friend." She tells me that her mother tends to be a bit anxious and at times depressed or sad. "She is much better now. She had more of those episodes when I was growing though." Her mom works outside the home as an administrative assistant at an insurance agency. "She started working there when I was in high school, and she was a stay-at-home mom when I was growing up." Her mother's parents are dead. Her grandmother died when Reilly was 13. She had a brain aneurysm and went to bed and never woke up, and "that was hard on us all." Her grandfather died last year. "He had a stroke and then died of pneumonia, and he was alert until the last day. It was sad, but I felt that he had lived a long life."

Reilly's father is 64 years old and runs a landscaping business. "He is very successful, has many people working for him." She describes that he tends to work all the time. "He has an office at home in addition to the store." He jogs every day. He has a history of hypertension and is on an antihypertensive agent. Being diagnosed with hypertension is what pushed him to start to take care of himself, according to Reilly. His mother died last year from colon cancer, and his father lives alone and is "in good shape for a man of 82."

Reilly has two siblings, a 32-year-old brother, Case, and a 29-year-old sister, Jennifer. Case is married to Madeline, and they have two children, 1 and 3 years old. Jennifer is gay and is in a committed relationship with Patty. They have no children. Reilly does not know of any emotional issues with her siblings. "Jennifer has had some tough times, but I am not sure if that is related to being gay. She was very depressed in high school, and then after she came out, she seemed to feel better about herself. My parents were a bit surprised when she told them, but they have really come along way. They are both very welcoming to Patty, and it is not a secret." Case is a "workaholic. It is a good thing he has a great wife. He is never home, and he is always going. He is a business executive and travels extensively."

Based on Reilly's shared family history, I knew I needed to delve deeper into what she meant by her mother's sad/depressed times and her father's somewhat hypomanic activities. These points of information stay in the forefront of my assessment process as we moved into Reilly's life event/stressor domain.

Reilly is the first of three children. She denied any significant events in her early childhood that made any lasting impact on her. She lived in a somewhat extended family model; her grandparents lived close by and were present in her life for many years. When she was 5 years old, Reilly moved with her family from a two-family rental house into the family house. She attended local public school, and for primary grades, she said, "I liked school. We could walk to my grammar school. It was before bussing in Boston, so many of the kids that I went to school with lived in my neighborhood." She remembers that her mom was at home and does not remember any significant changes when her siblings were born (she was 2 and 5).

As we moved into middle school memories, Reilly remembered having some difficulties with girlfriends and feeling left out of the gang. Her grades were "good" and "I played soccer and softball." She left grammar school after the 6th grade to attend 7th grade at the high school in the city that went from 7th through 12th grade. I had to take an examination to get into that school. It was an academically rigorous program, but I really wanted to go there because I knew it would help me get into a good college. Neither one of my parents went to college. Although they are successful in their own right, they really wanted me to go to college to pursue whatever I wanted to do. Education was very important in my house." The experience at the high school had many ups and downs for Reilly. "There were times when I would feel very focused, and then I would run out of steam. It was so frustrating. I would just feel so tired. I would know that it would go away. I just had to push through, and I would feel better. It seemed to be related to my period."

I asked Reilly how it was for her when her maternal grandmother died, as this occurred when she was 13 years old. "Oh that was terrible. No one had any idea. My mother was a mess, and she was so depressed. She was so close to her mother. I think she really had a major depression then, as well as being menopausal. She didn't get any help and just figured that time would take care of everything. Now I remember I ended up feeling like I had to take care of everything. She would be on the couch when I left in the morning and be there when I came home. My dad was busy, as usual, and he would come home at 7 p.m. and wonder where dinner was. They fought a lot during that time."

Although high school was academically a challenge, she described that socially it was okay. "Luckily Alison went to the same school. I think we helped each other get through. I had a group of friends that I hung out with. I was on the sports teams, and then I was in the gospel choir group. I had a few different boyfriends in high school but nothing exclusive or special. Well, there was one guy, Harry, I really loved him, but he ended up dating someone else over the summer after our senior year. That really was horrific. Isn't that funny? I almost didn't remember him, talk about Freudian!"

Reilly went away to college, which was "about 5 hours by car. It was difficult in the beginning as I was homesick, but then it was really great. I really liked college." I asked her whether she had any episodes in college of depression or times when she felt that she did not need a lot of sleep or felt agitated, irritable, or cranky. She remembered that she used to think, "and I still do think that I have seasonal disorder. I hate winter, and the transition into winter. I need the light." She also remembered episodes when she would pull "all nighters" to get work done and when she felt a bit "bitchy and cranky." "I figured I had PMS, as it would be around that time. I tried birth control pills, but they made me feel really irritable and witchy—not worth it, was my thought." Here was a key element in the assessment telling us that her brain did not tolerate the use of exogenous hormones, an important diagnostic indicator.

Reilly describes that she just pushed herself through those times, "writing it off to PMS or stress." She had one exclusive boyfriend for 2 years in college, "but that didn't work out." She describes some sadness when they broke up, but "it wasn't the end of the world." She finished college and sought a job back in Boston. "I really like this city." She lived with her parents for the first year after college. "That was okay, although we all had to go through an adjustment of my going out and I think of being an adult daughter. There were tense times, but fortunately, I had my own space, and my friends had apartments where I would stay on weekends to decrease the stress of coming home late on my parents."

Reilly secured a job after college in the financial arena and went to graduate school, part-time evenings, to secure her Master in Business Administration. Her special focus was finance. She had been with the same investment company for the past 10 years and planned to return to work as soon as she felt better. "This is horrific. What has happened to me? I wanted this baby. I am usually happy. What is going on?"

Reilly denied any major events since college that had caused her any difficulty. She met her husband, Owen, at graduate school. "He is such a nice guy. He is steady and calm, not like me, moody and irritable. He is worried about me and doesn't know what to do." She describes that they have had a nice life, although now that "I think about it there are times when I am a bit hyper, and he wonders what is going on, like when I decided that we needed to do the baby's room. I was a nut case. I was so focused on getting the right crib and the right stuff. He would just smile, and at the same time, I felt a bit out of control and wanted to scream at his, what appeared to me, as lack of attention to those details."

We then moved the focus of the assessment to the reproductive domain. Reilly had already given us some hints into her biochemical reactions to hormones. Reilly got her first period when she was 14 years old. She described some sense of irritability before her periods for most of her life. "I just figured I had PMS. Who doesn't?" She would experience some mood shifts during her cycle. "I really didn't focus on them. I just figured this too would pass." She had a regular cycle, about 30 days in length, moderate bleeding, and "really no problems." She did not like how she felt on oral contraceptives; thus, she had used a diaphragm and contraceptive creams and condoms for birth control methods. "I had very strong feelings that I did not want to get pregnant until I was ready."

She and Owen had been together for 4 years before they decided they were ready to start a family. "It was so funny. We decided we would eliminate the contraception, and I was pregnant the next month. It was a bit fast, but we adjusted." She describes that her pregnancy was fine. I asked her to elaborate on that and share with me how she felt in each trimester.

"Well, the first trimester was weird. I was tired and had significant morning sickness, but I never threw up. I felt a bit wired and irritable. There were times when I couldn't sleep, but I just figured it was pregnancy." Reilly described the second trimester as great. "I felt better. It was fun to have that baby inside my uterus. I loved talking to him, although I didn't know it was a him until he was born." The third trimester was also great, and "I worked until I went into labor."

The labor and delivery were uneventful. She described going into labor at work and calling Owen. They met at home and waited to see what happened. The contractions were coming about every 5 minutes. She called the doctor, and they were admitted to the hospital. "It was 7:00 p.m. I remember thinking that it was going to be a long night." The labor was uneventful. "I had an epidural, and that was nice. Then I pushed for about 2 hours, and out he came. We were so excited. I just cried and laughed. I couldn't believe I had done that and that we had a baby. Owen just smiled. He even had some tears in his eyes, too." The baby, Aden, weighed 7 pounds 5 ounces and was 21 inches long.

Reilly describes that her first day postpartum as wonderful. "I was so excited. I felt like I had conquered the world. I was the only woman who had given birth. He was beautiful, and I felt wonderful. All of my friends and family came to see us that night, and we all just laughed and joked. It was great." They were discharged from the hospital on day 2 postpartum, and then "I started to feel so down in the dumps. I cried at anything. I was so emotional. I felt edgy and anxious. I knew what I had to do, but there was a sense of overwhelming responsibility." Owen took that first week off from work, and they took care of Aden together. "The breastfeeding was so difficult in the beginning. I couldn't get the hang of it. He would cry, and I would cry. Finally, we figured it out, and I nursed him for about 3 months. I wasn't feeling that well, and I thought if I would stop nursing I would feel better, you know, have more energy. I just felt so tired and down in the dumps. It wasn't me, and I didn't know who this person was." As she had described before, she called her obstetrician, and he prescribed an anti-depressant for Reilly. The first one "had too many side effects," and this current medication, an SSRI agent, "I don't feel that great on." She is in therapy, which helps her because she has a place to talk. She feels that this is less "of a burden on Owen, but I want to go back to work. In my field, I have to be on my toes and able to focus, calculate, and process. I feel as though I am walking through a fog."

The assessment process was complete (see Figure 6.1). Now it was time to integrate the data and arrive at a diagnostic impression—what was

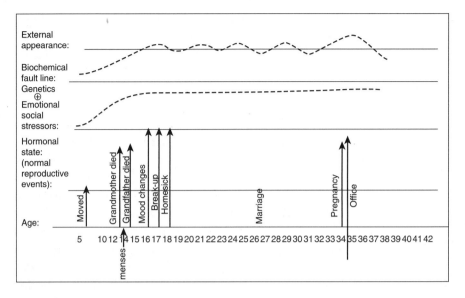

Figure 6.1   The Earthquake Assessment: Reilly
Sichel, D. & Driscoll, J. W.: *Women's Moods: What every woman must know about hormones, the brain, and emotional health.* 1999. By permission of HarperCollins Publishers, Inc., p. 100.

going on with Reilly's biology and psychology. She is presenting with depression as the primary symptom cluster, but significant or nodal events
in her history of a bipolar type nature cause one to consider a bipolar
diathesis or sensitivity or what Akiskal calls "soft bipolar" (Akiskal &
Mallya, 1987). She had a family history of a dad that had, what felt like,
workaholic tendencies. Was that hypomania? Her mother had episodes of
anxiety and depression. Reilly described agitation and irritability around
her menstrual cycle, times when she had a lot of energy, some mood
swings, a negative response to exogenous hormones, reactions to SSRI
agents, and alterations in her daily living secondary to the symptoms. My
thoughts were that she had a bipolar sensitivity. Currently, she was being
treated with an SSRI agent at a therapeutic level, but she was not feeling
any better. Thus, I decided to augment the antidepressant with a mood-
stabilizing agent to see whether we could get some significant results and
that would help with the differential diagnosis.

I discussed the biochemistry of the process with Reilly and explained
that I felt that based on her symptoms postpartum and what sounded like
some mood swings in high school and college, especially around her menstrual cycles, that we would need to add a mood stabilizer. We discussed
the use of Depakote, lithium, and lamotrigine. I went over the potential

side effects and the use of each agent, the blood levels, and so forth. Reilly liked the sounds of the Lamotrigine the best because it had no weight gain or sexual side effects. We discussed the process of starting the dosing at a very low level; then we would increase the dose very cautiously. I informed Reilly of the significant side effect called Steven Johnson Syndrome, which can occur if the dosing is too rapid. She would need to pay attention to the development of any rashes, and if she found one, we would refer her to a dermatologist to ascertain whether it was a lamotrigine rash or something else, especially if the medication was helping her. We would not touch the SSRI agent that she was currently taking, as I do not like to change too many things at one time, as you can never be sure of what caused what. Reilly was also having a difficult time getting to sleep; she describes that she worries about everything. I decided to use an atypical neuroleptic, in this case olanzapine, to quiet her brain at night so that she could get to sleep. This agent is a mood stabilizer and has a more rapid onset of action than the lamotrigine. In this way we could get her brain to get some sleep while we slowly increased the lamotrigine.

We then discussed, developed, and collaborated on her NURSE Program (Sichel & Driscoll, 1999), which was as follows:

Nurse Program

- **Nutrition and needs:**
  - Reilly needed to increase her protein intake at meals and eat small, frequent meals with protein snacks.
  - She would increase her water intake to 8 to 10 8-oz. glasses per day.
  - She would continue a daily multivitamin.
  - She would add omega-3 fatty acids (3,000 mg), 500 mg of vitamin C, and 400 IU of vitamin E to her daily supplements.
  - She would add calcium supplements, as she does not consume dairy products, and we hope to avoid osteoporosis before menopause.
  - Lamotrigine (Lamictal) (12.5 mg per day for 5 days and then increase to 25 mg per day for 5 days) was added.
  - Olanzapine (Zyprexia) (2.5 mg tablet) at bedtime was added.
  - The SSRI agent was prescribed by the obstetrician.
  - She felt that she did not need any additional help around her house, as her partner was really an active co-parent and would take care of lots of things so that she could rest more.

- **U**nderstanding: Reilly was in a therapy relationship with a psychologist and felt that that relationship was positive and helpful. She signed a release so that I could contact her therapist to collaborate in Reilly's care. I would also be contacting and informing her obstetrician of the medication additions and my coming on board as a team member. I also suggested the use of a journal as another strategy to in essence "download her feelings and concerns" in a safe, nonjudgmental space.
- **R**est and relaxation:
  - We discussed Reilly's sleep hygiene program:
    - Going to bed at same time every night and waking at the same time every morning
    - Bedtime rituals that might help get her in the mood to go to sleep, for example, a warm bath, focused relaxation, a massage from her husband, etc.
  - Meditation strategies, breathing exercises, and yoga

- **S**pirituality:
  - Reilly described a strong sense of spiritual connection with her religion. She was raised Catholic and felt that prayer was very helpful to her.

- **E**xercise:
  - Thirty minutes per day at least 5 days per week: walking in the morning before Owen went to work and going back to the gym that she used to belong to before the pregnancy, as they had a day care center and Reilly knew the women at the gym.
  - Taking the baby out in the stroller and walking briskly in the middle of the day if she was feeling well, as exercise would increase the endorphin secretion, which can help with mood.

Reilly felt that she understood the plan of care, and we arranged to meet again the next week. Until we arrived at the therapeutic level of medication based on her responses, we would be meeting weekly. Reilly was aware that she could call me with any questions or concerns, and that I considered nothing to be unintelligent. We talked a lot about what had gone on using the Earthquake Assessment, and she seemed to feel comfortable with the plan. I did want her to call me the next day to tell me how she did taking the olanzapine for sleep as well as just to check in. Her therapist and obstetrician were called later that day.

The next day Reilly called, "I slept like a rock. Owen was on call if Aden woke up, but I slept so well. I feel so different this morning." I suggested that she continue the olanzapine for a few more nights so that we could give her brain some good restorative sleep as well as time for the lamotrigine to kick in. She agreed to that and we would see each other the next week.

At the next visit, Reilly described feeling more directed and clearer. "I feel like I am coming out of the fog. It is so much better." She was beginning to think that she could go back to work at some time. "The office told me that I could come back whenever I felt ready to. They are holding my position. I have great day care. Owen's sister runs a day care, and she has a spot for Aden. I feel good about that. I am just afraid that I am not going to continue this upward momentum."

This is the hard part of the care plan, developing trust that the positive healing will continue. There is always fear that the symptoms will return, especially because they have in the past. There is a tendency for some exacerbation of symptoms during the late luteal phase of the menstrual cycle. Thus, we would be monitoring that over the next few months. Sometimes that is a clue from the brain that we need to increase the mood-stabilizing agent. We discussed the unique titration for her biochemistry and the necessity to stay on medications for at least a year. Then we would re-evaluate her situation. It is my clinical impression that she may need to stay on medications for a longer period, and we spoke of that but decided to just focus on the present.

As it turned out, Reilly did very well on 75 mg of lamotrigine and 2.5 mg of olanzapine premenstrually for a few nights. We discontinued her antidepressant at about 1 month after the initiation of the lamotrigine. She is aware that we need to plan to work together regarding the use of medications in pregnancy or the weaning from medications before another conception. No significant data are currently available regarding these medications and pregnancy, although the beginning research is looking good. They both agreed to use adequate contraception.

References

Akiskal, H. S. (1996). The prevalent clinical spectrum of bipolar disorders: Beyond DSM-IV. *Journal of Clinical Psychopharmacology*, 16(Suppl), 4S–14S.

Akiskal, H. S., & Mallya, G. (1987). Criteria for the "soft" bipolar spectrum: Treatment implications. *Psychopharmacology Bulletin*, 23(1), 68–73.

Akiskal, H. S., Bourgeois, M. L., Angst, J., Post, R., Moller, H., & Hirshfeld, R. (2000). Re-evaluating the prevalence of and diagnostic composition within the broad clinical spectrum of bipolar disorders. *Journal of Affective Disorders*, 59, S5–S30.

Altshuler, L. L., Cohen, L. S., Moline, M. L., Kahn, D. A., Carpenter, D., Docherty, J. P., & Ross, R. W. (2002). Expert consensus guidelines for the treatment of depression in women: A new treatment tool. *MentalFitness*, 1(1), 69–83.

American Psychiatric Association. (2000). *Diagnostic and statistical manual of mental disorders* (4th ed.). Text Revision. Washington, DC: Author.

Amsterdam, J. D., & Brunswick, D. J. (2003). Antidepressant monotherapy for bipolar type II major depression. *Bipolar Disorders*, 5(6), 388–395.

Angst, J. (1998). The emerging epidemiology of hypomania and bipolar II disorder. *Journal of Affective Disorders*, 50(2–3), 143–151.

Benazzi, F. (1999). Gender differences in bipolar II and unipolar depressed outpatients: A 557-case study. *Annals of Clinical Psychiatry*, 11(2), 55–59.

Benazzi, F. (2001). Sensitivity and specificity of clinical markers for the diagnosis of bipolar II disorder. *Comprehensive Psychiatry*, 42(6), 461–465.

Bowden, C. L. (2001). Strategies to reduce misdiagnosis of bipolar depression. *Psychiatric Services*, 52(1), 51–55.

Calabrese, J., Suppes, T., Bowden, C. L., & Al, E. (2000). A double-blind, placebo-controlled, prophylaxis study of Lamotrigine in rapid cycling bipolar disorder. *Journal of Clinical Psychiatry*, 61, 841–850.

Colaizzi, P. (1978). Psychological research as the phenomenologist views it. In R. Valle & M. King (Eds.), *Existential phenomenological alternatives for psychology* (pp.48-71). New York: Oxford University Press.

Driscoll, J. W. (2004). *The experiences of women living with bipolar II disorder.* Doctoral Dissertation, University of Connecticut, unpublished.

Dunner, D. L. (1992). Differential diagnosis of bipolar disorder. *Journal of Clinical Psychopharmacology*, 12(1 Suppl), 7S–12S.

Dunner, D. L. (2003). Clinical consequences of under-recognized bipolar spectrum disorder. *Bipolar Disorders*, 5(6), 456–463.

Dunner, D. L., & Fieve, R. R. (1974). Clinical factors in lithium carbonate prophylaxis failure. *Archives of General Psychiatry*, 30, 229–233.

Ghaemi, S. N., Hsu, D. J., Soldani, F., & Goodwin, F. K. (2003). Antidepressants in bipolar disorder: The case for caution. *Bipolar Disorders*, 5(6), 421–433.

Goldberger, N. R., & Truman, C. J. (2003). Antidepressant-induced mania: An overview of current controversies. *Bipolar Disorders*, 5, 407–420.

Hadjipavlou, G., Mok, H., & Yatham, L. N. (2004). Pharmacotherapy with bipolar II disorder: A critical review of current evidence. *Bipolar Disorders*, 6, 14–25.

Hirschfeld, R. M. A., Bowden, C. L., Gitlin, M. J., Keck, J., P. E., Perlis, R. H., Suppes, T., et al. (2002). Practice guidelines for the treatment of patients with bipolar disorder (revision). *The American Journal of Psychiatry*, 159(4 Suppl), 1–50.

Kendell, R., Chalmers, J., & Platz, C. (1987). Epidemiology of puerperal psychosis. *British Journal of Psychiatry*, 150, 662–673.

Kessler, R. C., McGonagle, K. A., Zhao, S., Nelson, C. B., Hughes, M., Eshleman, S., et al. (1994). Lifetime and 12-month prevalence of DSM-III-R psychiatric disorders in the United States: Results of the National Comorbidity Survey. *Archives of General Psychiatry*, 51, 8–19.

Legato, M. J. (2002). *Eve's rib: The new science of gender-specific medicine and how it can save your life.* New York: Harmony Books.

Leibenluft, E. (Ed.). (1999). *Gender differences in mood and anxiety disorders: From bench to bedside* (Vol. 18). Washington, DC: American Psychiatric Press.

Leibenluft, E., Fiero, P.L.,& Rubinow, D.R. (1994). Effects of the menstrual cycle on dependent variables in mood disorder research. *Archives of General Psychiatry, 51,* 761-781.

Lewis, F. T. (2004). Demystifying the disease state: Understanding diagnosis and treatment across the bipolar spectrum. *Journal of the American Psychiatric Nurses Association,* 10(3), S6–S15.

Mitchell, P. B., Wilhelm, K., Parker, G., Austin, M. P., Rutgers, P., & Malhi, G. S. (2001). The clinical features of bipolar depression: A comparison with matched depressive disorder patients. *Journal of Clinical Psychiatry, 62,* 212–216.

Post, R. M., Leverich, G. S., Nolen, W. A., Kupka, R. W., Altshuler, L. L., Frye, M. A., et al. (2003). An evaluation of the role of antidepressants in the treatment of bipolar depression: Data from the Stanley Foundation Bipolar Network. *Bipolar Disorders,* 5(6), 396–406.

Sichel, D. A., & Driscoll, J. W. (1999). *Women's Moods: What every woman must know about the hormones, the brain, and emotional health.* New York: William Morrow Publishers.

Simpson, S. G., Folstein, S. E., Meyers, D. A., McMahon, F. J., Brusco, D. M., & DePaulo, J. R. (1993). Bipolar II: The most common bipolar phenotype? *American Journal of Psychiatry,* 150(6), 901–903.

CHAPTER 7

POSTPARTUM ANXIETY DISORDERS

Little is known about sex-related features or mechanisms associated with anxiety disorders. The onset or exacerbation of an anxiety disorder or a panic disorder is not uncommon during the postpartum experience. The ovarian hormones and their metabolites have bioactive effects and can contribute to the occurrence or susceptibility of women to panic (Yonkers & Kidner, 2002). In this chapter, panic disorder and obsessive compulsive disorder (OCD) with postpartum onset are addressed.

Panic Disorder with Postpartum Onset

Health care providers need to differentiate between postpartum depression and postpartum panic disorder. Postpartum depression has been used as a catchall phrase for other postpartum mood and anxiety disorders. Women may be misdiagnosed with postpartum depression when in reality they are suffering from postpartum onset of panic disorder. Each of these mood and anxiety disorders has its own distinctive symptoms and unique potential for disrupting the newly formed family unit, and each requires different treatment.

In 1988, Metz and Sichel described panic disorder presenting for the first time in the early postpartum period. Sichel, the second author, encountered 11 mothers with panic disorder for the first time shortly after childbirth. Fisch (1989) described five cases of panic disorder presenting for the first time in the postpartum period in Israel. Sholomskas et al. (1993) examined whether the onset of panic initially during the first 3 months postpartum was a coincidental occurrence. Sixty-four mothers who had delivered at least one child and had been diagnosed with panic disorder were interviewed by telephone. Seven women (10.9%) met these criteria for postpartum onset of panic disorder compared with the expected percentage of 0.92%. The mean onset of postpartum panic was at 7.3 weeks postpartum.

In my concept analysis of panic (Beck, 1996), fieldwork included studying women with postpartum panic to obtain qualitative data for further analysis. In focusing on empirical indicators of panic, the fieldwork revealed that all of the DSM-IV's (American Psychiatric Association, 1994) indicators of panic were experienced by the mothers. Additional indica-

---

Criteria for Panic Attack:

"A discrete period of intense fear or discomfort, in which four (or more) of the following symptoms developed abruptly and reached a peak within 10 minutes:
  1. Palpitations, pounding heart, or accelerated heart rate
  2. Sweating
  3. Trembling or shaking
  4. Sensations of shortness of breath or smothering
  5. Feeling of choking
  6. Chest pain
  7. Nausea or abdominal distress
  8. Feeling dizzy, unsteady, lighthearted, or faint
  9. Derealization (feelings of unreality) or depersonalization (being detached from oneself)
  10. Fear of losing control
  11. Fear of dying
  12. Paresthesias (numbness or tingling sensations)
  13. Chills or hot flushes" (APA, 2000, p. 432)

Reprinted with permission from the *Diagnostic and Statistical Manual of Mental Disorders*, Copyright 2000. American Psychiatric Association.

tors of panic were hysterical crying, distortion regarding time, and painful feelings in the head.

The postpartum period appears to be associated with the worsening of panic symptoms (Beck, 1998; Cohen et al., 1996). Eleven percent to 29% of women with panic disorder reported an onset during the postpartum period (Wisner, Peindl, & Hanusa, 1996). Women with a history of mild panic symptoms have experienced worsening of those symptoms in the postpartum period. This worsening characteristically occurs within the first 2 to 3 weeks and may be accompanied by symptoms of depression.

Mitral valve prolapse and hyperthyroidism, which have been associated with panic disorder, occur more frequently in women; thus, it is imperative that these disorders be concurrently ruled out (Lohr, Kamberg, Keeler, & Ak, 1986). Premenstrual hormonal changes may play a role in panic disorder, which would implicate the role of ovarian hormones in vulnerability to anxiety and panic in the postpartum period (Metz & Sichel, 1988). The association of reproductive hormonal changes in women with panic disorder needs further exploration, as biological sex differences in vulnerability may influence the prevalence of panic disorder in women. Fluctuating levels of sex hormones may influence the neurotransmitter system or other physiologic parameters and change the threshold for symptom management (Yonkers & Kidner, 2002).

In response to limited research on this postpartum anxiety disorder, I conducted a phenomenologic study to describe women's experiences with panic during the postpartum period in order to help clinicians better differentiate postpartum panic disorder from other postpartum mood and anxiety disorders (Beck, 1998). Through interviews with mothers diagnosed with postpartum panic disorder, six themes emerged that described the essence of the mother's experience.

Theme 1: The terrifying physical and emotional components of panic paralyzed women, leaving them feeling totally out of control.

During panic attacks, women endured distressing physical symptoms such as chest pain, heart palpitations, shortness of breath, dizziness, tightening of the throat, and tingling in extremities. One woman attempted to capture the physical sensation that occurs during panic: "It was like somebody injected Coca-Cola into my veins. Between the bubbles and the caffeine, everything was just rushing." Women's sight and hearing were also affected by their panic. Women describe incidents of blurry vision and amplified sounds that occurred during a panic attack.

One can appreciate just how distraught women became while enduring panic attacks from the detailed description provided by a Cambodian woman.

> *My body always feels hot. I feel hot tears, hot flashes, and most of the time, I feel hot inside of my head. I feel shaky. It seemed that every time I closed my eyes, something broke out in my head. It is like the noise, the sound of my computer. I feel pain. It starts from the bottom of my feet up to my head. I feel like the blood is moving up to my head faster and faster. My face is hot. I fear the pain—the muscle spasms over my heart. I start to feel, "Am I going to have stroke?" It is getting worse and worse. It spreads. I fear that it might damage my heart.*

As panic worsened and women lost all sense of control in their lives, some had suicidal thoughts. One mother painfully divulged,

> *I always knew it was crazy, but I needed to do it. I would write to my baby almost as if I knew I was going to die, which is morbid. I would write what I felt about him and how much I loved him. I think because in the back of my mind I was always afraid that I might kill myself [quietly weeping].*

Theme 2: During panic attacks, women's cognitive functioning abruptly diminished, whereas between these attacks women experienced a more insidious decrease in their cognitive functioning.

In the midst of a panic attack, women were terror stricken that they were losing their minds. An eerie sense of impending doom indulged women during panic attacks. Women repeatedly said that their thinking was irrational. One put it this way: "My cognitive functioning went out the window." Catastrophic misinterpretations of their physical symptoms were made while experiencing panic. This was illustrated by the following quote:

> *During the panic attacks, I would have chest pains and shortness of breath. I thought that I was having a heart attack and that I was going to die. I remember having gone to the emergency room a few times just to have someone tell me that I was okay. They said that I was abusing the emergency room. It was just for an emergency!*

Between panic attacks, women were not able to trust their minds or judgments because they were so consumed with worry over the panic. The fear of the panic was distracting in their everyday lives. Aware of her diminished cognitive functioning, one woman began to videotape her child talking and singing because as she explained,

When he is 15, I want to listen to his voice when he was a baby so that
I can hear it when I am normal. Because I am not sure now that when
I hear him babbling and going that what I am even hearing is normal.

Theme 3: During the panic attacks, women feverishly struggled to maintain their composure, leading to exhaustion.

When panic suddenly hit, women frantically strove to " keep the panic down" and to maintain their composure. Some women fled outdoors for a breath of fresh air. Others were compelled to keep moving because sitting or standing in one place was inconceivable. While experiencing a panic attack, women would desperately try to talk themselves out of the panic to no avail. Women repeatedly reported that after an attack was over, total exhaustion set in. A lot of energy was expended trying to hide panic from others and pretending that all was well.

Theme 4: Because of the terrifying nature of panic, preventing further panic attacks was paramount in the lives of the women.

As one woman painfully stated, "My life was completely consumed with panic prevention, which was motivated mainly by my own hypervigilance to appear normal and not to disgrace my family." After enduring panic attacks for varying periods, women sought to discover specific panic triggers particular to their own lives. Certain times of the day would trigger panic attacks in some women. For example, one said that at sunset she would feel like everything was closing in on her, and often panic would suddenly hit her. For another, when she awoke, panic attacks would occur. Being confined indoors, such as in a church or a meeting room, would trigger panic attacks in other women. At times, being away from their babies would trigger a panic attack. During certain phases of a woman's menstrual cycle, panic attacks would occur more often. For instance, one woman discovered that her panic occurred only between the time that she ovulated and the end of her period. Some women realized that their panic attacks were more prevalent when they had a lot of commitments and were really stressed. Another trigger for some women was being alone, especially when their minds were not occupied.

Some women had an insatiable desire for information about panic disorders, hoping to discover a remedy for their panic. The terror involved in panic attacks drove all of the women to seek professional psychiatric help. Desensitization was one strategy employed by some women to alleviate panic. For example, before her daughter's christening, one mother made an appointment with the priest to rehearse the ceremony.

Theme 5: As a result of recurring panic attacks, negative changes in women's lifestyles ensued—lowering their self-esteem and leaving them to bear the burden of disappointing not only themselves but also their families.

Fearing the onset of a panic attack, some women drastically curtailed their activities. Some, for example, no longer flew in airplanes, went skiing, or even drove their own cars. Tormented by panic attacks occurring when they left the safety of their homes, some women secluded themselves as much as possible.

When some women could no longer tolerate the panic on their own and they finally agreed to take medication that their psychiatrists prescribed, one of the most agonizing changes in their lives occurred: They had to stop breastfeeding. Self-esteem plummeted as their panic caused drastic changes in their lives. Women believed that they had become totally incompetent. They had lowered their standards for accomplishments. One woman poignantly said this:

> The personal disappointment is the hardest part. I had such great
> aspirations for myself, but now I wonder. Sometimes I could cry that
> I can't do things that other people do. The disappointment is over-
> whelming to me that I used to be this really unbelievably function-
> ing person. When I was in college, I could do anything until I had a
> baby and the panic started.

Mothers anguished over their belief that they had repeatedly let their families down because of their panic. The heart-wrenching disappointment some women experienced in themselves as a result of their panic is quite apparent in the passage that follows. One mother could not bear to attend story hour and said,

> I can't believe I could be so disappointed in myself. I couldn't
> bear that my son was losing out. I don't know. I guess I really just
> wanted him to enjoy story hour like all other kids, but when I got
> home I just cried. I cried for hours cause I felt like I was a bad mother.
> I was just so disappointed in myself, but we never went back.

Theme 6: Mothers were haunted by the prospect that their panic could have residual effects on themselves and their families.

Even though the women were recovering from their panic, they were afraid it would never be completely gone. Women were vehement that no matter how long it had been since they had recovered from their panic, the piercing memories would be permanently imprinted in their minds. The following passage illustrates this point:

> *I can hardly drink a cup of coffee without flashing back on the panic.*
> *Even though it was how coffee makes you have that rush, that*
> *feeling will drive me crazy to the point now that I don't drink coffee*
> *or tea or any coke with caffeine in it. I know it's going to take some*
> *time, but it's just terrible. Terrible doesn't even describe it. It is ab-*
> *solutely unbelievable. The panic is the worst thing imaginable.*

Mothers were fearful that their panic would traumatize their children. One mother painfully recounted her fear:

> *I was so afraid that I would leave a permanent mark on my son—*
> *the way I was would rub off on him. I just wished for his life that he*
> *could do well in spite of me somehow. Some mothers wondered if*
> *they had been so preoccupied and consumed with the panic that*
> *they missed their children's cues. Had their children needed them*
> *they were not able to notice?"*

Reprinted with permission from Beck Postpartum Onset of Panic Disorder. Image: *Journal of Nursing Scholarship,* pp. 133–134 (1998).

Treatment

Selective serotonin reuptake inhibitors (SSRIs), monoamine oxidase in-hibitors (MAOIs), and tricyclic antidepressants have all demonstrated efficacy in the treatment of panic disorder (Sheehan, 1999). The SSRI agents are effec-tive in panic symptoms, even when symptoms of depression are not present. High-potency benzodiazepine medications, such as lorazepam, alprazolam, and clonazepam, are also effective antipanic medications. The classes of SSRIs, MAOIs, tricyclic antidepressants, and benzodiazepines are associated with similar rates of improvement (60% to 70%) in panic symptoms (Pigott, 2002). Buspirone and other medications with primary serotonergic effects do not appear to be more effective than placebo for panic disorder (Bell & Nutt, 1998). The adjunct use of cognitive behavioral therapy is also useful.

Case Study

Marissa is a 29-year-old woman who is 4 weeks postpartum with her first child. She is currently complaining of "anxiety" that seems to get worse. "Now I feel like I am having panic attacks all through out the day, I am afraid to go outside of the house for fear that I will have an episode and something bad will happen." As we sat in my office, I shared that I would be asking her questions to assess how her brain had arrived at this place.

Marissa is the second child of four: two brothers and a sister. Her mother is 55 years old and works as a laboratory technician in their local hospital, and her father, 56 years old, is a math teacher in the public school system. "He is thinking about retirement soon." Her mother "is an anxious mess, but has never gotten any help, although she does have her one to two glasses of wine every night." She describes that her father is "the calm one" and that he is the one she calls on if she has a problem. "My mom makes mountains out of molehills!" Her parents have no significant medical illnesses or any proclivities toward any. Her brothers and sister are all alive and well. "My older brother is in recovery from alcohol use and is doing well. He lives in Georgia with his wife and their two kids." Her younger brother is living near their parents and is in a relationship with a woman; they are considering marriage in the future. "He is a bit anxious and worries about things. He has been in therapy for about 2 years. He is working on his doctorate in counseling psychology." She is close to her sister, "although that was not always the way. She and I are 22 months apart. I aligned more with my older brother, so we have only become closer as we have gotten into our adulthood." Her sister is living in New Jersey, and she is married with no children and works as a teacher in the primary school in her town. She is anxious and tends "to make lists about everything, and recently, she told me that she has been having a rough time premenstrually and that she was contemplating going to see someone for that."

When Marissa thinks about her life, she does not remember any significant events that were bad. As she was contemplating her life, we learned that she had moved from Philadelphia to Connecticut when she was in the fourth grade and that at that time she remembers having a lot of stomach aches when she would go to school. "I didn't like taking the school bus. It would make me feel sick." Her mother would drive her to school, and eventually, that went away. "Now that I think of it, I did not do very well with any big change. We moved when I was in the eighth grade. I really hated that. I had to go into a new school, and I knew no one. It was horrific. I remember that my stomach hurt all of the time, and I just wasn't very happy. It took me a while before I was involved in some of the school activities and felt like I had any friends. I remember really being angry with my parents even though I never told them. They were happy that we were in a bigger house and thought that we all would be happy too. It was a rough time for me, and then I went to a new high school. That wasn't as hard because my brother was there, and I knew his friends. It was an easier adjustment." She went away to college "about 2 hours from home" and majored in psychology. She describes that she met her husband while she was in graduate school. "He was getting his master's in business administration. We got married after we both graduated. He took a job up here in the Boston area, and I was able to get a job in one of the hospitals."

When I asked her how that transition was, she describes that she was excited to be marrying Danny, as he is really "the love of my life." He is very nurturing, and they are "able to talk about everything. In fact, he is the one that kept pushing me to call you when we got your name from my nurse-midwife. He is very worried about me and would be here if he could, but he had a major meeting today. I told him I would be fine. Can he come into another visit?" I told Marissa that Danny was welcome to come for a session so that he could share his thoughts and concerns; then I would be able to educate him about postpartum mood and anxiety disorders and discuss things that he can do to help her. I feel that postpartum mood and anxiety disorders affect the whole family; thus, the more that I can educate and inform, the better the care plan is supported and followed. As we were collecting her history, I began to see that she indeed had experienced some tremors in her biochemistry when she described the anxiety experiences during transitions in her life (see her Earthquake Assessment chart, Figure 7.1). Based on the theories of allostatic loading (McEwen, 1998), one could surmise that as Marissa got older and experienced more events in her life that her ability to recover from transitional events would take longer and perhaps not be as biochemically efficient. I moved to the area of Marissa's reproductive history to finish the assessment process.

I asked her about the onset of her first menstrual period (menarche). She had her first period when she was 13 years old. "It came when I was eighth grade. I remember it happened at school that first month, and I didn't know what to do. I ended up going to the nurse, and she had sanitary pads in her office. My mother had prepared me. She read that book with me—you know the one about changing bodies." She did not have any problems with her menstrual cycle. "It came regularly and really didn't get in the way of my living in any way. The thing I do remember was trying to use tampax for the first time. That was horrible. I almost passed out. I was at a party and someone gave me one to try. Eventually I learned how to use them, but that took a long time."

Marissa did not remember any significant anxiety symptoms around her menstrual periods. "I do remember though when I started on birth control

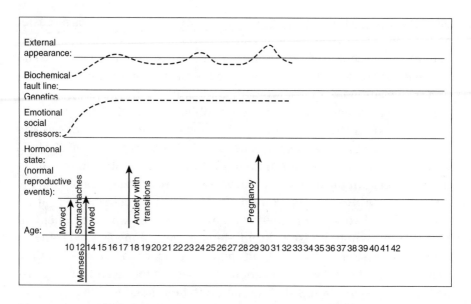

Figure 7.1 The Earthquake Assessment: Marissa
Sichel, D. & Driscoll, J. W.: *Women's Moods: What every woman must know about hormones, the brain, and emotional health.* 1999. By permission of HarperCollins Publishers, Inc., p. 100.

pills in college that it took a few different trials for me to find the right doses of hormones. I had headaches and nausea with a lot of them. I really can't remember the names of them now." This was her first pregnancy, and she and Danny had planned for this pregnancy. "We felt that we were ready to have a baby—little did I know I would feel this way."

"I stopped the birth control pills, and then about 3 months later we were pregnant." She described the first trimester as a time of "some anxiety" as well as nausea. "Although I rarely threw up, I was very tired though." She told me that she spent time pondering: "Is this real? I am going to have a baby. Will the baby be healthy, and will I be a good mother?" She had these thoughts and then would talk to herself and remind herself that she was healthy and that she and Danny were in it together. They would do fine. Marissa used a form of self-talk to help quiet and calm her anxious thoughts; thus, I knew that I wanted to build on the coping strategy that she already had. The second trimester was fine with no big issues or concerns. The third trimester was a time of increased anxieties and concerns. "We took the childbirth classes, and that was when I started to get more anxious. I was hearing more stories from friends and acquaintances regarding their birth experiences. Some of them were a bit hairy."

She practiced her breathing strategies, and Danny would practice with her at night in their bed. "We were ready. I think we were both nervous about how would we know when we had to go to the hospital. I have a wonderful nurse-midwife, and she was and still is so supportive to me and to him, too." Marissa worked until she delivered the baby and planned to stay out of work for 3 months.

She described the labor and delivery experience, as well as the first day after the baby was born. My goal in this assessment piece is to ascertain any symptoms of hypomania during that first 24-hours postpartum. The contractions began while she was at work. "It felt like a backache; it would come and go, but it wasn't uncomfortable. I found myself just walking around and rubbing my back. I didn't have to use any breathing strategies at all. I did call my nurse-midwife and shared with her my symptoms, and she said that was sounding like something was happening and that she was indeed on call that night, which I was very glad to know." Marissa went home from work, and she and Danny spent a quiet night watching television. As the evening went on, the contractions seemed to get stronger and were now in the front of her uterus. Eventually, they were coming every 5 minutes, and she found that she was getting a bit "anxious." Thus, they called the nurse-midwife. They were told to come to the hospital. They arrived at the hospital at about 11:00 p.m., and Marissa was admitted and found to be 4 centimeters dilated. They settled into the labor room and walked the halls for as long as they could. Marissa had intended to have an unmedicated childbirth and was happy that she was able to do that. "I found that the breathing was very helpful, and Danny was great. He was right there all of the time. I was fully dilated by 6 a.m., and I pushed for about 1 hour. It was an amazing experience and when she was born. I just sobbed. Danny cut the cord, and he had tears dripping down his cheeks. We just laughed and cried. She was and is beautiful." Marissa had given birth to a lovely little girl named Monica. The baby was in her arms in my office peacefully sleeping.

At this point, Marissa began to cry, "Jeanne, it was downhill from that point." She could feel the anxiety begin to rise, as it was time to take care of Monica and attempt to breastfeed her. "I was so anxious that I would be able to do it. I had read all of the books, and my nipples were fine; however, I was a mess. She latched on right away and sucked the way that they said she was supposed to, but I wasn't confident of anything. She nursed regularly. They told me that she was doing well, but I kept thinking to myself, "How could she be getting enough milk from me as I am so nervous. I didn't tell anyone what my concerns were. I was a good patient. I did share with Danny that I was a bit worried about the nursing, but he was reassuring and told me that we would take one day at a time." They were discharged from the hospital on day 2 and went home to their apartment, just the three of them. "My mother wanted to come up and visit, but I told her to not come until the weekend so that we could have some time alone as a family. To be honest with you, Jeanne, I knew that she would make me more nervous in that she did not nurse her babies. She was already asking me how I would know if the baby got enough food."

The first few days postpartum were as would be expected. Marissa shared with me that she and Danny laughed and cried together. He was home for the days after the birth, and they learned to care for their daughter, Monica. "The breastfeeding was going fine, I guess, but I was worried about her gaining weight. The visit to the pediatrician at week 2 was critical to me. Danny took that day off, and she had gained almost 2 pounds! The baby was born at 7 pounds 6 ounces, was discharged at a weight of 6 pounds 15 ounces, and at that visit had weighed about 8 pounds. I was thrilled." The focus of the anxiety shifted now from the breastfeeding to the idea of going out alone with the baby.

"Oh, I forgot to tell you. My mother did come up that weekend, and she stayed for 2 weeks. That was helpful in that Danny went back to work, and my mother made the dinner, did the laundry. On the whole, she was very supportive. It was just little things that she did that I would just watch and not say anything about. She changed the baby and would put baby oil all over her head. She would tell me that that was what she was taught, to keep the scalp moist. She also did not think that we should pick her up as soon as she cried, little things like that." Danny and Marissa would debrief the visit in the evening when he came home from work. It appeared that the mother's visit was good in some ways, but according to Marissa, "I was more anxious about performance, in that how did my mother know and I knew nothing about my baby. I began to doubt myself inside, but I didn't talk about it. I was worried that something would happen when she left, and I had to go out with Monica alone."

According to Marissa, the anxious feelings did not go away but rather began to feel as though the anxiety was with her all of the time. "I just felt a bit jumpy, a bit disconnected at times, like I was having a cold sweat. My stomach was a bit unsettled. I would be on the couch and think of things to do. Then I would get panicky and just count the hours until Danny came home." She disclosed that once he was home she could relax and knew that she was not alone. The first panic attack took place when she went out one day to visit her colleague from work for lunch at her home. "I got Monica in the car seat. We started to drive, and my heart started to beat quickly. I felt tightness in my chest. I felt lightheaded. I pulled over to the side of the road and did some cleansing breaths and talked to myself; it calmed down. I got to my friend's house, and to be honest with you, I did not want to leave; not saying anything to anyone, I knew I had to be strong and get back in the car drive home. It happened again, and when I got home, I just started to cry." The panic attacks were coming with greater frequency of late, and that is what led her to call her nurse-midwife and then call me.

Currently, she was experiencing anxiety symptoms all through the day and having panic attacks two to three times per day. She feels that she is out of control and terrified that one of these attacks is going to cause her to drive off the road or that she will be so anxious that something will happen to Monica. In a review of the systems, we assessed her nutritional status, sleep behaviors, exercise history and current regime, lochia flow/status, and feelings of support networks. In sitting with Marissa, I felt that she was experiencing an anxiety/panic disorder with an exacerbation in the postpartum period. She had some vulnerability for anxiety from her genetics and her response to transitions and change. Thus, I told Marissa that I thought she had an anxiety disorder but that we wanted to make sure that her thyroid functioning was normal. We needed to talk with her primary care provider about any cardiac history of murmur or mitral valve prolapse. Marissa said that she had never experienced the heart palpitations until this experience and had not been told that she had any mitral valve issues by her primary care physician (PCP). I described the physiologic changes that can occur after the birth of the baby that can alter the vulnerable brain biochemistry and that she had some history of anxiety prepregnancy. At that time, cognitive strategies such self-talk and breathing strategies had helped her; however, now those techniques may need a bit of biological help, such as medication, to help quiet her anxiety.

We began to develop her NURSE Program (Sichel & Driscoll, 1999).

- **N:** Nutrition and needs: This aspect of the care plan would now include the use of antianxiety agents to help to quiet the anxiety response in her body. I would prescribe Klonopin 0.5-mg tablets and suggested that she take one-half tablet at bedtime and then in the morning and see how she felt. She could take up to 1 mg per 24 hours with minimal effect on the breastfeeding and her infant (Altshuler et al., 2002; Birnbaum, 1999). We would try that first and see how she responded to that; if that medication worked, we would leave that as the medication treatment plan, but if she found that that dose was not holding her symptoms at bay, we would initiate the use of an SSRI agent, which is approved for use with breastfeeding and anxiety disorders. We went over her nutrition, ascertaining her protein, fluid, and vitamin intake. I suggested that she begin omega-3 fatty acids, in addition to 400 IU of vitamin E and 500 mg of vitamin C to work as antioxidants for the fatty acids.

- **U:** Understanding: I suggested that she come to meet with me once a week for a few weeks for supportive psychotherapy and medication management. It is important for her to have a place to share her fears/concerns and to work through this experience so that she could move forward in her own parental growth and development as well as personally. We talked about how postpartum is an opportunity to rethink and restrategize coping strategies as well as a time to work through personal issues and concerns. Often when looking at one's child, one begins to remember childhood events and memories that need to be verbalized and processed. Often, women will hear the voice of their mother come through from their childhood in statements they had vowed they would never use when they had children. The therapy relationship is a safe place to process that information and to feel that it was important for them to witness and process. There is a degree of grieving that goes on in this experience, as one mourns who she used to be to begin to accept who she is becoming, someone's mother and/or father.

- **R:** Rest and relaxation: The rest and relaxation had to do with her sleep patterns/rituals. Marissa felt that after she got to sleep she was okay. It was the anticipatory stage of the sleep process that she had a hard time with. "That is when my worries come forth and I think about them and the next day." We discussed the rituals of getting to bed at a regular time, potentially using a bottle for Danny to feed Monica, keeping the television out of the bedroom, writing in a journal express thoughts, using relaxation tapes, and so forth.

- **S:** Spirituality: This was not a concern for Marissa. "I pray all the time to the Blessed Mother to take care of Monica, Danny, and me. I do have faith, Jeanne, that this will all be okay. It is just hard to stay focused."

- **E:** Exercise: Marissa had not had her postpartum checkup yet and was still experiencing some discharge vaginally, although the bright bleeding had ended. It was now more of a dark color and seemed to be getting less every day. She was beginning to go out for walks with the baby but waited until Danny was home to go with her. She had limited her trips in the car, as that was a place that the panic attacks really started, and she is anxious that that will happen again. (She had had one when she had come to my office today.)

I asked her whether she had any questions. She did not. Thus, we scheduled a meeting for the next week. She knew that she could call me with any question and concerns, and that I considered nothing to be un-intelligent. She packed up Monica, smiled through her tears, and said, "Thank you. I'll see you next week."

The next week Marissa, Monica, and Danny came to the appointment. Danny was happy to be there and said that he felt that she was doing better. Marissa agreed, although she had found that she did not really feel totally calm and relaxed. She felt that she would have moments but that the anxiety would return. At this time, we decided to add a low dose of sertraline (Zoloft), 12.5 mg per day. She would continue the clonazepam (Klonopin) in addition to the Zoloft. Over the next few weeks, we would increase the sertraline and then begin to decrease the Klonopin use. I went over side effects of the SSRI, as well as the research pertaining to the use of SSRI agents and breastfeeding infants. We went over her NURSE program.

Over the next few weeks, she continued to increase her sertraline dose to 50 mg, and she told me that she was feeling much calmer and that the anxiety was not present at all. Now she was concerned about decreasing the Klonopin. She was currently taking 0.5 mg at bedtime; thus, we began with a taper of the Klonopin to 0.25 mg at bedtime for a week, and then 0.125 mg, and then nothing. That taper was successfully completed. She did have to go up to 100 mg of sertraline and in therapy worked on issues of responsibility (as the oldest daughter) and her pervasive anxiety regarding what other people thought about her and how she was learning to feel authentic in herself and her personal relationship with self. I continued to see Marissa for a year, and then she felt that she was ready to come off the medications and think about another child. She tapered off the sertraline at 12.5 mg per menstrual cycle and agreed to stop meeting. She plans to call me when she gets pregnant with her second child so that we can develop the care plan, anticipating the postpartum anxiety, and be prepared if it did indeed occur again.

Obsessive Compulsive Disorder (OCD) with a Postpartum Onset

Diagnostic Criteria for OCD

A. Either obsessions or compulsions:

Obsessions as defined by 1, 2, 3, and 4:

1. Recurrent and persistent thoughts, impulses, or images are experienced at some time during the disturbance as intrusive and inappropriate and cause marked anxiety or distress.
2. The thoughts, impulses, or images are not simply excessive worries about real-life problems.
3. The person attempts to ignore or suppress such thoughts, impulses, or images or to neutralize them with some other thought or action.
4. The person recognizes that the obsessional thoughts, impulses, or images are a product of his or her own mind (not imposed from without as in thought insertion).

Compulsions as defined by (1) and (2):

1. Repetitive behaviors (e.g., hand washing, ordering, checking) or mental acts (e.g., praying, counting, repeating words silently) that the person feels driven to perform in obsession or according to rules that must be applied rigidly.
2. The behaviors or mental acts are aimed at preventing or reducing distress or preventing some dreaded event or situation; however, these behaviors or mental acts either are not connected in a realistic way with what they are designed to neutralize or prevent or are clearly excessive.

B. At some point during the course of the disorder, the person has recognized that the obsessions or compulsions are excessive or unreasonable. This does not apply to children.

C. The obsessions or compulsions cause marked distress; are time consuming (take more than 1 hour a day); or significantly interfere with the person's normal routine, occupational (or academic) functioning, or usual social activities or relationships.

D. If another Axis I disorder is present, the content of the obsessions or compulsions is not restricted to it (e.g., preoccupation with food in the presence of an eating disorder, hair pulling in the presence of Trichotillomania, concern with appearance in the presence of body dysmorphic disorder, preoccupation with drugs in the presence of a substance use disorder, preoccupation with having a serious illness in the presence of hypochondrias, preoccupation with sexual urges or fantasies in the presence of a paraphilia, or guilty ruminations in the presence of major depressive disorder).

E. The disturbance is not due to the direct physiologic effects of a substance (e.g., a drug of abuse, a medication) or a general medical condition.

Specify if:
With poor insight: if, for most of the time during the current episode, the person does not recognize that the obsessions and compulsions are excessive or unreasonable" (American Psychiatric Association, 2000, pp. 462–463).

Reprinted with permission from the *Diagnostic and Statistical Manual of Mental Disorders*, Copyright 2000. American Psychiatric Association.

Postpartum OCD

OCD affects about 3% of the general population, and more than half of that population is women (Brandes, Soares, & Cohen, 2004). The incidence of postpartum OCD is unclear, as it has been largely understudied. Pregnancy and postpartum may represent a time of increased vulnerability for the initial emergence of OCD or for significant worsening in women with pre-existing OCD (Pigott, 2002). When undiagnosed and untreated, postpartum OCD can cause suffering and dysfunction in both the patient and her family. The maternal child attachment and interaction may be interrupted, and adverse developmental, cognitive, and behavioral effects may develop in the newborn.

The cause of OCD is unknown, although serotonin dysfunction has been suggested (Barr, Goodman, & Price, 1993; Pigott, 2002). The etiology of postpartum onset OCD is unknown. The acute onset may be due to the dramatic, rapid fall in the female hormones of estrogen and progesterone, resulting in a dysregulation of the serotonin, which then interacts with any predisposition to mental disorders (Sichel, Cohen, Dimmock, & Rosenbaum, 1993; Williams & Koran, 1997). Another hypothesis regarding etiology, suggested by McDougle et al. (1999), is the rapid increase in oxytocin to a high level near the end of pregnancy and during the postpartum period, which may trigger an exacerbation or the onset of OCD. They felt that oxytocin may play a role in the pathogenesis of unwanted and recurrent sexual thoughts or images that are common in women who are not pregnant with obsessive disorder (McDougle, Barr, Goodman, & Price, 1999).

In 1990, OCDs in association with childbirth were first described (Buttolph & Holland, 1990). Eight of 27 mothers with OCD reported to have the onset of their OCD symptoms during the early postpartum period. Women are at increased risk of developing OCDs during the postpartum period (Altshuler, Hendrick, & Cohen, 1998; Buttolph & Holland, 1990). In 1993, Sichel et al. reported on 15 women who presented with OCD after childbirth (mean of 2.2 weeks postpartum). The symptoms involved with this OCD were obsessions to harm the infant, elevated generalized anxiety, and a disruption in the relationship between mother and infant. The symptoms were limited to mothers' intrusive obsessive thoughts of harming their infants, but there were no compulsive rituals. The mothers' predominant source of distress was their intrusive thoughts. All of the mothers experienced some degree of avoiding their infants for fear of harming them. None of the women were psychotic. None of the mothers ever acted on their intrusive thoughts. Sichel et al. (1993) stressed the need for clinicians to distinguish between OCD and postpartum psychosis, in which a mother is at risk of harming her infant.

Existing data (Epperson et al., 1995; Maina, Albert, Bogetto, Vaschetto, & Ravizza, 1999) suggested that the onset of OCD is common in the postpartum period. Postpartum OCD exacerbation is fairly consistent in women with preexisting OCD. Most studies have reported that 20% to 30% of females with OCD will experience a significant postpartum worsening in OCD symptoms (Altshuler et al., 1998; Buttolph & Holland, 1990; Sichel et al., 1993; Sichel, Cohen, Rosenbaum, & Driscoll, 1993). It is also evident that there are differential characteristics in the presentation of postpartum onset of OCD, with respect to the presence or absence of compulsions and the contents of the obsessions and/or compulsion as compared to non-postpartum related OCD (Brandes et al., 2004).

Williams and Koran (1997) reported that 7 of the 24 mothers (29%) with preexisting OCD who had completed pregnancies shared that they had exacerbation of their OCD symptoms during the postpartum period. Nine of the 24 mothers (37%) with preexisting OCD also reported postpartum depression. Williams and Koran stressed the need for careful evaluation after delivery of mothers with OCD because they are at risk for developing postpartum depression.

Recent life events, specifically the role of delivery and postpartum events, have been examined as triggers to OCD onset (Maina et al., 1999). Retrospectively, Maina et al. using a case-controlled design investigated 68 patients (33 of whom were females) who had been diagnosed as having OCD without concurrent major depression. The birth of a live child was the only life event during the 6 to 12 months before the onset of OCD that was significantly different for the OCD women as compared with the comparison women. Eight women (24% of the female patients) mentioned the birth of a child as a precipitating event and reported that their new onset of OCD began within the first 4 weeks after delivery. OCD women were more likely than the comparison women to report higher rates of obstetric complications. Mothers with postpartum OCD had significantly higher rates of aggressive obsessions to harm their infants than the comparison women.

When postpartum OCD is undiagnosed and subsequently untreated, significant suffering and dysfunction can happen not only for the patient but also for the family and its development. Interruption in the mother–infant bond occurs secondary to the mother's fear that she may act on her thoughts, and this may affect the cognitive–behavioral development of the infant.

Assessment

Assessment is critical, as this disclosure tends to be associated with shame and guilt on the part of the new mother. The clinician needs to ascertain the frequency, duration, and intensity of the thoughts. The woman needs to be asked whether she has had the feeling that she would act on her thoughts, and if a positive response is given, a need may exist for psychiatric referral and intervention sooner rather than later. Most women will describe the thoughts but then go on to tell the clinician that there is no way that she would act on the thoughts. In fact, you usually hear the elaborated behavioral plans that the woman had developed to avoid the situations in which the thoughts might occur, like having all of the knives, sharp objects, andirons from the fireplace taken out of the house and locked away in an undisclosed location. One woman shared with Jeanne that she left her house at 6:30 a.m. and drove around until it was an appropriate time to visit her friend. She felt that as long as she was not alone with her child, that her child would be safe. "I just needed another adult around, although I never told them why."

Most women with postpartum OCD are terrified to share their thoughts with anyone because they fear that their child will be taken away from them in addition to the shame, guilt, and blame. Education and reassurance are mandatory for postpartum OCD so that women receive appropriate care and do not have to suffer in silence.

Postpartum depression or concurrent major depression must be excluded during the assessment, as there is a comorbidity factor with OCD and depression. Blood work needs to be done to ascertain any physiologic abnormalities: anemia, thyroid dysregulation, and such. It is critical to differentiate between "normal" worry about the new baby versus obsessions. Obsessions should be differentiated from ruminations in major depression (Brandes et al., 2004).

The woman must realize that she is not losing her mind and that her obsessions are thoughts and not deeds. Be sure to assess for psychosis, which is a rare complication of postpartum. Postpartum psychosis is frequently considered to be a manifestation of bipolar disorder or a manifestation of major depression with psychotic features (Arnold, Baugh, Fisher, Brown, & Stowe, 2002; Gold, 2002).

Treatment

As with any treatment plan, the patient must be informed and educated regarding the disorder, the potential etiology as reported by the state of the science, and the treatment choices along with risks and benefits as needed. Treatments include psychotherapy, cognitive–behavioral therapy, and pharmacologic methods. Attention must be paid to the lactational status of the woman and her involvement in the decision making based on what compliments her values and beliefs. As a clinician, I (Jeanne) strongly endorse some form of psychotherapy if medications are to be used as a treatment method. It is imperative for the woman have a place to process the occurrence of this disorder, mourn the loss of her expectations to accept the reality of this current experience, and to forgive herself for the thoughts that were not under her control. The therapy relationship is critical to the healing of postpartum mood and anxiety disorders, as there is the facilitation of her development as a mother/person, and she has a safe place to establish trust and disclose her fears, shame, and concerns.

Treatment with SSRI agents is very effective in most cases. According to Brandes et al. (2004), large, randomized, double-blind, placebo-controlled studies have demonstrated the efficacy and tolerability of the SSRIs fluoxetine (Tollefson et al., 1994), sertraline (Greist et al., 1995), paraoxetine (Zohar & Judge, 1996), fluvoxamine (Goodman et al., 1989a), citalopram (Koponen et al., 1997; Marazziti et al., 2001; Montgomery, Kasper, Stein, Bang Hedegaard, & Lemming, 2001), and clomipramine (DeVeaugh-Geiss, Katz, Landau, Goodman, & Rasmussen, 1991; Montgomery, Montgomery, & Fineberg, 1990; Montgomery et al., 2001; Thoren, Asberg, Cronholm, Jornestedt, & Traskman, 1980) in treatment for the general population. Recent data on the use of venlafaxine for the treatment of OCD are encouraging (Albert, Aguglia, Maina, & Bogetto, 2002; Ananth, Burgoyne, Smith, & Swartz, 1995).

The specific data on the efficacy of the SSRIs and clomipramine in the treatment of postpartum OCD are limited; however, the data on nonpostpartum women and their efficacy suggest their use with postpartum episodes.

I (Jeanne) have found that it is best to begin the dosing at low doses and gradually increase over time until the symptoms disappear or are minimal. Antianxiety agents (benzodiazepines) are often needed to augment the antidepressants.

Clinically, many women are able to wean from the antidepressants after about a year of treatment. The weaning process is as gentle and slow as getting on the medications. It seems to help with the process by bringing down the dose at each menstrual cycle. Women have reported that they sometime have a premenstrual return of anxiety, and an occasional thought will pop into their mind; however, they seem to be able to cope with those episodes as they feel more in control of the experience. Some women have not been able to wean from the medications as the symptoms surface and cause them anxiety at a certain level of medication; thus, I bring the dose up to the level that covers them biochemically, and the thoughts do not resurface. No formula exists regarding who this will happen to versus who it will not happen to.

OCD seems to be a recurrent problem, and women may experience exacerbations in subsequent pregnancies and postpartum experiences. In light of this preventive anti-OCD medication, therapy is initiated very quickly after birth. This is where the relationship between the patient and the clinician is critical. A care plan needs to be developed from the onset of the pregnancy to help the woman feel supported regardless of which scenario is played out, as we really cannot predict, and there are limited studies pertaining to panic disorder and OCD in the pregnancy and postpartum period. For information regarding psychopharmacologic treatments and breastfeeding, see the appendix.

Early and aggressive treatment of OCD in the postpartum period is critical in order to minimize the dysfunction to the woman and her family.

Case Study

Lisa is a 28-year-old married woman who came into my office for an evaluation. She made this appointment at the recommendation of her obstetrician, as she has been having severe anxiety symptoms since the birth of her baby. Lisa came into my office, carrying her baby in the infant seat, sits on the couch, and begins to cry. I smile gently at Lisa and ask her to share what she is feeling. She tells me that she doesn't know what is wrong with her and that she cannot believe that she is here. "I don't think I am crazy, but something is wrong."

It is not uncommon for the patient to feel even more anxious about contacting a psychiatric care provider based on the stigmatization of psychiatric illnesses and care, especially for a postpartum woman who feels that all she did was have a baby! It is essential to pay attention to this early relational issue so that connection is promoted and empathic mutuality is felt by the patient from the provider. It is usually the call that is made after all other avenues of care have been initiated without results, so there is also an element of self-esteem loss. "I can't even handle having a baby. What is wrong with me?" This feeling is often the self-disparagement that comes through when the woman sits across from me. My priority is to establish the relationship, to provide safety and support during the interaction, and to normalize the exaggerated postpartum response. Postpartum is a major physiologic crisis that can precipitate multiple physiological responses in addition to physiologic changes of lactation!

I encouraged Lisa to share with me the events of her postpartum experience to date, and then we would move into the additional information that I would need for the Earthquake Assessment. Lisa was 12 weeks postpartum. She described that this was a planned pregnancy. "We were very excited about the pregnancy. We had tried for about 5 months after we stopped using condoms."

"We have been married for 5 years, and we just felt we were ready to start a family. We bought a house a year ago, and it just seems right. Anyway, the pregnancy was fine. I was nauseous in the early weeks and a bit nervous. I just figured that was normal. I continued to work. I work in a bank as a cashier. I was tired at the end of the day, but not bad. We took childbirth classes in the third trimester, and I really wanted to try to deliver the baby without any medications. The labor was long, about 22 hours, but I was energized when I could push. Then she was born. It was amazing.

Harry cut the cord, and we both were amazed with how perfect she was."
At this point, I asked Lisa to describe the first day after the birth of the
baby and how the past 12 weeks had been.

"Well, that first day I was just so excited and at the same time scared of
taking care of her. She was so tiny and so perfect. She weighed 6 pounds
5 ounces and was just perfect. She has the biggest eyes. That first day I was
trying to learn how to breastfeed her. She seemed to know exactly what to
do. I was a bit nervous about whether she would get enough milk. That is
a continual concern for me, even though she has gained weight beautiful-
ly from breast milk. I still worry. Anyway, I was anxious about her sleeping
position, especially with my worry about sudden infant death syndrome. I
would make sure that she was on her back or her side and really didn't let
her get on her tummy at all. I was worried about her position, whether she
was too warm, too cold, and if I held her head correctly. I was especially a
mess if anyone came to visit. I worried that they might have germs and that
she would get sick. I feel as though I am just anxious all of the time and
worried about her safety."

At this point, I waited until Lisa took a pause and kindly asked her
whether she ever had any strange, funny, weird, or scary thoughts about
something happening to her daughter Michaela. She looked at me quickly
and said, "How did you know that? Are you going to report me?" I asked
Lisa who she thought I was going to report her to. She thought that I would
have to call the Department of Social Service because she was having
horrific thoughts of something bad happening to her daughter. I softly
asked Lisa to share with me the thoughts that she was having and what she
did when she had the thoughts.

"I am so afraid that I am going to drop her on the floor, and then at times,
I have had these really bad thoughts that I could harm her with a pencil or
a fork. One time, I even imagined that her small fingers could be cut like
niblets in a corn can. I feel so bad, Jeanne. I am not a bad person. Why am
I thinking this? You asked me what I do when I have the thoughts. You are
going to think I am nuts, but I have had Harry put all of the knives, sharp
kitchen utensils, and anything that makes me anxious in the basement. He
just looks at me when I tell him they are making me nervous. I think he just
humors me because I have told him that I am afraid something might
happen to Michaela. He tries to be reassuring, but I think he wonders what
is going on. I mean, I have always been an anxious person but never had
bad thoughts before." Lisa is crying while she is talking to me and rubbing
her daughters back as she burps her gently.

I feel that Lisa is having obsessive thoughts that are basically rooted in her issues of safety and concern; however, the basic concern gets exaggerated, and the fear is that the thought will become the deed. This is a type of anxiety disorder that is called postpartum obsessive thought disorder. It is treatable, and we can work on her feeling better. I share with her that I am not sure of the rate of occurrence with this disorder but that I have heard the same symptoms from many women once they feel safe enough to reveal to me their "terrible thoughts." I also shared with her that it had been my experience that women with this disorder do everything they can to keep their babies safe and secure. I then informed Lisa that I needed to secure additional information from her regarding her family history, her life, and her reactions to that life so that we could begin to put together the puzzle pieces and figure out how these symptoms presented themselves at this time in her life—postpartum.

We began with family history. Lisa described that her mother was a very anxious woman and that she was always checking in on her to make sure that Lisa was doing all right. "Sometimes she drives me crazy in that she calls two times or more a day. I know she thinks she is supportive, but that makes me more nervous." Lisa's mother had birthed two children, one son and Lisa. They were 3 years apart. "I don't know what her postpartum experiences were like. I just know that she is afraid to go anywhere without my Dad. She really is nervous when I think about it." She describes her father as "the calm and patient one." Her dad "takes good care of mom." He is still working as an insurance broker at the same firm he has for the past 25 years. He plays golf and cards with his buddies at the club regularly. She denies any mood or anxiety disorders in her father or on his side of the family. Her mother, as stated earlier, appeared to live with an anxiety disorder, maybe even panic with agoraphobia. Lisa's maternal grandparents were both dead. Her grandfather died of pancreatic cancer when Lisa was 22, and her grandmother died that same year of an aneurysm. She thinks that her maternal grandmother was also a "nervous Nelly. I remember my mother commenting about her mother and her nerves." Lisa's brother is younger than she and is living in Chicago. "He seems to have inherited my dad's gene. He is calm and patient. We are very close. He calls every day to see how I am and whether there is anything he can do to help me. He helps me just by calling. I could never tell him the thoughts that I am having. Oh, Jeanne, am I crazy? Would I hurt my baby?"

I reassured her that we were going to work together to help her feel better and calm her anxieties and concerns. We then moved on to her life event history. I asked her whether she could remember significant events in her life and to describe her reaction to those events if she could recall. We began with the early years of her life. Lisa did not remember any significant events in her very early childhood. She did remember grammar school. "I was a bit anxious. I didn't want to leave my mom when I went to first grade. I had to take a bus and that made me scared. I remember worrying that it would be in an accident." She described that grammar school was really uneventful except "when I think back, I was nervous a lot of the time. I would hum songs to make me feel more relaxed. Isn't that funny I remember that now?" High school presented a new scenario for the presentation of anxiety and what started to sound a bit like some obsessive thoughts. "I was a nervous student. I was always studying hard, worried about the test and the grade. I was in the drama club and did have some significant roles in the plays, but it was such hard work for me to quiet my anxiety. As I said, I hummed a lot. I don't remember if it was out loud or just to myself. Isn't that funny, now I remember that." Lisa did well in high school and went away to college in the Washington, DC area. She describes severe homesickness for the first semester at college. She did get into a counseling relationship at college. "I went to the student counseling services and saw a therapist for about 6 weeks. She helped me learn some new strategies to deal with my anxieties and my fears and concerns. I did some cognitive work with thought stopping and assessing and changing my cognitive distortions. That helped a lot, and I still use those skills today; however, they are not holding me now."

During college, she met Harry, and they began dating during her junior year. "It was love at first sight. He is just the most centered, loving man. I am so lucky. That makes this even harder. He knows that I have a propensity for anxiety, but this has been so extreme and scary. Harry is feeling at a loss. He doesn't know what he is supposed to do. Should he be firm or supportive with me?" This is a common issue between the couple, as the partner is trying to help her "out of it" and thinks that if he or she doesn't feed into their partner's anxieties then maybe it will stop. On the other hand, they see their partner in such distress that it is hard to not be supportive and at the same time frustrated and maybe even angry. As one partner said to me one time, "This is not the woman that I married. She is a mess. She won't even go out of the house, and she won't let anyone help with the baby, including me. I have had it. I wonder if this marriage is going to last." As you can imagine, the couple may indeed need some support and some therapy to help the healing process after the woman is feeling that her anxiety is under control and she has more energy to work on the relationship with the other versus needing to focus on the self.

Lisa was married after she graduated from college. She took a job in a bank and has been happy working there. Harry works for an insurance company and continues to sit for certification examinations that advance him in his profession. He had taken his last exam during her last month of pregnancy and will not be focusing on another test until next year. "He decided to hold off on that exam so that he would be more available to us this year."

We then moved into the domain of Lisa's reproductive life experiences. Lisa recalls that she experienced her first menstrual period when she was about 13 years old. "I remember I was at my aunt and uncle's house on the Cape when I got my period. My cousin is 2 years older than me, so I asked her whether she had any sanitary products. Luckily, she had some pads. It took me a while to learn how to use tampons." She did remember that she had had what seemed like more anxiety before her period started and usually feels an increase in anxiety premenstrually. "I tried the birth control pills when I was in college, but I felt like I was jumping out of my skin. We have used condoms and are religious about using them. I have to tell you it was nice not to use them when we were trying to conceive. Now we are back to them again."

She describes that her periods are regular, and she does not experience any bad symptoms such as cramps or headaches premenstrually—"just the anxious feeling." As she had shared with me early in our session, this was a planned, wanted pregnancy, and she did experience some exacerbations of anxiety and worry during her pregnancy. That brought us to the current situation. I felt that Lisa was experiencing an exacerbation of her previous anxiety disorder with obsessive thoughts. It is thought that the obsessive thoughts exhibited during the postpartum experience are due to the cascade of brain hormones that trigger maternal–infant attachment. Sichel and Driscoll (1999) described that these obsessive thoughts may be due to the oxytocin and an overshooting of the maternal hormone that promotes protection and safety. It is normal for a new mother to identify potential threats that may harm her infant and to move to protect the baby. In postpartum obsessive thought disorder, those thoughts regarding danger and protection get started but do not find their way to the ultimate conclusion of protection. Rather, the thought of harm keeps occurring repeatedly in the mother's brain, and then she begins to experience anxiety that she may act on the thoughts. She cannot stop the thoughts. It is like the needle getting stuck in the old vinyl records of the 1970s.

The incidence of this disorder is uncertain, as we are just hearing about it from women more and more because of the changes in the information regarding postpartum illnesses in the lay literature and professional literature (Brandes, 2004). It was important to educate Lisa about this disorder so that the shame and blame could be lessened and hopefully not occur. This is a biological situation, and when we treat the brain with the right medication, the anxieties and thoughts should decrease and hopefully disappear. What then occurs is that women will talk about their memories of the thoughts, and this is the work of the psychotherapy during the healing process.

The treatment of postpartum obsessive thought disorder generally includes the use of the SSRI agents or Anafranil, a tricyclic antidepressant that is particularly serotonergic. The decision about which medication to use is based on family history, sensitivities, presenting symptoms, and feeding choice. Anafranil is a relatively safe agent to be used with breast-feeding; however, as a tricyclic agent, it does have the potential for side effects of postural hypotension, and the catecholamine effects of dry mouth, constipation, and perhaps weight gain. I generally begin at low doses and move up gently over time. I also use antianxiety agents such as Klonopin or Ativan to augment the effects of the SSRI agents, and they act quickly so that there are some responses while the antidepressants are taking their time to work.

I shared with Lisa what my diagnostic conclusion was and then described for her the plan of care that I would be recommending and how we would be working together with our goal of wellness and enhanced maternal–child relationships, intrapersonal relationship, and interpersonal comfort (see Figure 7.2). The NURSE Program (Sichel & Driscoll, 1999) that was developed for Lisa included the following:

- **N: Nutrition and Needs:**
  - Eat small frequent meals with adequate protein intake at each meal, including yogurt, cheese, tuna fish salad, cold cuts of roast beef, and turkey.
  - Drink 8 to 10 8-oz. glasses of water per day.
  - Continue maternal vitamins, add 3000 mg of omega-3 fatty acids, 400 IU of vitamin E, and 500 mg of vitamin C.
  - Medications:
    - Begin 0.25–0.50 mg clonazepam (Klonopin) twice a day to decrease anxiety and promote sleep. The baby slept through the night currently, and Harry had been giving her a bottle of pumped

breastmilk regularly; thus, that behavior was encouraged. Lisa was encouraged to go to bed after the feeding at about 9 or 10 p.m., and if the baby woke before 4 or 5 a.m., Harry would feed the baby pumped breastmilk this week. (The plan would be re-evaluated at each weekly session.)

- Anafranil (clomipramine) 25 mg orally at hour of sleep (HS) for 4 days then increase to 50 mg per day (reevaluate at next session, blood level to be obtained in 2 weeks). Anafranil was chosen, as it is okay to use with breastfeeding and is a good medication to quiet her thoughts and anxiety. SSRI agents can also be used with this disorder, whereas the serotonergic nor-epinephrine reuptake inhibitor (SNRI) agents have limited data to support safety with lactation. With obsessive disorders, the level of serotonergic reuptake agent is usually higher than with depression alone.

- **U:** Understanding: I shared with Lisa that postpartum onset of ob-sessive thought disorder responds well to the use of medications but that psychiatric medications take a longer time to reach therapeutic

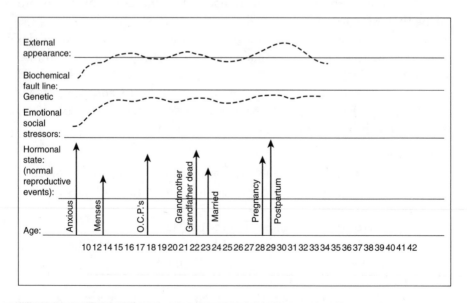

Figure 7.2   The Earthquake Assessment: Lisa
Sichel, D. & Driscoll, J. W. *Women's Moods: What every woman must know about hormones, the brain, and emotional health.* 1999. By permission of HarperCollins Publishers, Inc., p. 100.

range, so her symptoms would be decreasing slowly over time. It is like a gentle lifting of the curtain, moving from black to dark grey to grey to light grey to white. It is a frustrating process because in our culture we are so used to the quick-fix approach with medication—take an ibuprofen and the headache goes away quickly. She would need to understand that the mechanisms of the antidepressant medications take longer. Lisa had a clear sense of the use of cognitive strategies to change the thoughts in her head; thus, we went over thought-stopping strategies, self-talk methods, diversion tactics, as well as using journaling and/or talking to someone. She was encouraged to call me with any concerns/questions/issues, as I felt that nothing was silly and that it was not uncommon to need a bit of reassurance during this healing process. I also shared with Lisa that I feel strongly about concurrent psychotherapy with the psychopharmacotherapy, as it is a place to talk about feelings, issues, and concerns as she moves through motherhood, and that she will have a place to mourn, grieve, and work through her healing as the thoughts decreased and hopefully went away.

- **R: Rest and Relaxation:** She would be taking the Klonopin initially to help treat the anxiety symptoms and to help her rest at night. She could begin with 0.25 mg at HS, or if that didn't help her to increase to 0.5 mg at HS. If she felt that she was having a lot of anxiety in the day, she could take 0.25 mg of Klonopin after awakening and then again about 6 to 8 hours later. It is recommended that for a breastfeeding mother, the dose of Klonopin be kept to 1 mg per day (Altshuler et al., 2002).
- **S: Spirituality:** Lisa did not practice a formal religion at this time but did believe in God and shared with me that she prayed every day. I encouraged her to use prayer as a form of meditation and to use the breathing strategies that she had learned in her childbirth classes.
- **E: Exercise:** Lisa was 12 weeks postpartum and had just begun to return to the gym. She found that it was easier to go for a walk in the morning before Harry went to work, and she also took the baby out in the carriage when the weather was nice outside. I encouraged her to continue her walking and to try to do some fast walking to break a sweat and to encourage the secretion of the endorphins that help with mood.

I summarized our visit for Lisa and asked her whether she had any additional questions. We scheduled an appointment for the next week. I encouraged her to bring Harry, if he could come, so that he could be part of the care plan, as postpartum emotional problems do affect the whole family, and I wanted him to know that he was part of the treatment plan. Lisa said that she felt better and that in a strange way it was nice to know that she was not crazy and that we would be able to help her feel better. She understood that she had a propensity toward this disorder with her history of anxiety and her genetic hard wiring being vulnerable secondary to her mother's symptoms. She put Michaela back into the infant carrier and off they went.

I saw Lisa weekly for about 3 months, and we continue to meet currently about every 3 weeks. We increased her Anafranil to a dose that quieted her symptoms, and her blood levels put her in therapeutic range. She exhibited a few side effects such as constipation, which was treated by increasing fluids and adding more fruit to her diet. She continued nursing her daughter and discontinued the Klonopin about 3 weeks into the treatment plan. In the therapy, she was able to become more aware of how her anxiety presented itself, and she developed coping strategies to deal with issues and concerns in her life.

Generally, I keep women on the medication treatment plan for a minimum of 1 year after we have achieved the therapeutic dose. When they verbalize their desire to get off the medications, my weaning plan is done by going down a dose at each menstrual cycle. It takes a bit longer, but clinically I have seen less rebound and exacerbation of symptoms. With obsessive disorders, a small percentage of women in my practice cannot get off the medication at the 1-year mark; thus, I have tried it at different intervals from that point on. Some are able to discontinue the medications at some point, whereas others are maintained on a lower dosing ritual.

References

Albert, U., Aguglia, E., Maina, G., & Bogetto, F. (2002). Venlafaxine versus Clomipramine in the treatment of obsessive-compulsive disorder: A preliminary single-blind, 12-week, controlled study. *Journal of Clinical Psychiatry*, 63, 1004–1009.

Altshuler, L., Hendrick, V., & Cohen, L. S. (1998). Course of mood and anxiety disorders during pregnancy and the postpartum period. *Journal of Clinical Psychiatry*, 2, 29–33.

Altshuler, L. L., Cohen, L. S., Moline, M. L., Kahn, D. A., Carpenter, D., Docherty, J. P., et al. (2002). Expert consensus guidelines for the treatment of depression in women: A new treatment tool. *Mental Fitness*, 1, 69–83.

American Psychiatric Association. (1994). *Diagnostic and statistical manual of mental disorders* (4th ed.). Washington, DC: Author.

American Psychiatric Association. (2000). *Diagnostic and statistical manual of mental disorders* (4th ed.). Washington, DC: Author.

Ananth, J., Burgoyne, K., Smith, M., & Swartz, R. (1995). Venlafaxine for treatment of obsessive-compulsive disorder. *American Journal of Psychiatry, 152*, 832.

Arnold, L. M., Baugh, C., Fisher, A., Brown, J., & Stowe, Z. N. (2002). Psychiatric aspects of the postpartum period. In A. H. Clayton (Ed.), *Women's Mental Health: A comprehensive textbook* (pp. 91–113). New York: The Guilford Press.

Barr, L. C., Goodman, W. K., & Price, L. H. (1993). The serotonin hypothesis of obsessive compulsive disorder. *International Clinical Psychopharmacology, 8*, 79–82.

Beck, C. T. (1996). A concept analysis of panic. *Archives of Psychiatric Nursing, 10*, 265–275.

Beck, C. T. (1998). Postpartum onset of panic disorder. *IMAGE: Journal of Nursing Scholarship, 30*, 131–135.

Bell, C., & Nutt, D. (1998). Serotonin and panic. *British Journal of Psychiatry, 172*, 465–471.

Birnbaum, C.S., Cohen, L.S., Bailey, J.W., Grush, L.R., Robertson, L.M., & Stowe, Z.N. (1999). Serum concentrations of antidepressants and benzodiazepines in nursing infants: A case series. *Pediatrics, 104*, e11.

Brandes, M., Soares, C. N., & Cohen, L. S. (2004). Postpartum onset obsessive-compulsive disorder: Diagnosis and management. *Archives in Women's Mental Health, 7*, 99–110.

Buttolph, M., & Holland, A. (1990). OCD in pregnancy and childbirth. In W. Minichiello (Ed.), *Obsessive-compulsive disorders: Theory and management* (pp. 89–97). Chicago: Year Book Medical.

Cohen, M. Z., Sichel, D., Faraone, S. V., Robertson, L. M., Dimmock, J. A., & Rosenbaum, J. F. (1996). Course of panic disorder during pregnancy and the puerperium: A preliminary study. *Biological Psychiatry, 39*, 950–954.

DeVeaugh-Geiss, J., Katz, R., Landau, P., Goodman, W., & Rasmussen, S. (1991). Clomipramine in the treatment of patients with obsessive-compulsive disorder: The Clomipramine Collaborative Study Group. *Archives in General Psychiatry, 48*, 730–738.

Fisch, R. (1989). Postpartum anxiety disorder. *Journal of Clinical Psychiatry, 50*, 268–269.

Epperson, C. N., McDougle, C. J., Brown, R. M., Leckman, J. F., Goodman, W. K., & Price, L. H. (1995). OCD during pregnancy and the puerperium. *American Psychiatric Association New Research Abstract*, NR112, 84.

Gold, L. H. (2002). Postpartum disorders in primary care: Diagnosis and treatment. *Primary Care, 29*, 27–41.

Goodman, R., Price, L. H., Rasmussen, S. A., Mazure, C., Fleischmann, R. L., Hill, C. L., et al. (1989a). The Yale-Brown Obsessive Compulsive Scale: I: Development, use, and reliability. *Archives in General Psychiatry, 46*, 1006–1011.

Greist, J., Chouinard, G., DuBoff, E., Halaris, A., Kim, S. W., Koran, L. M., et al. (1995). Double-bind parallel comparison of three dosages of sertraline and placebo in outpatients with obsessive-compulsive disorder. *Archives in General Psychiatry, 52*, 289–295.

Koponen, H., Lepola, U., Leinonen, E., Jokinen, R., Penttinen, J., & Turtonen, J. (1997). Citalopram in the treatment of obsessive-compulsive disorder: An open pilot study. *Acta Psychiatry Scandinavia*, 96, 343–346.

Lohr, K. N., Kamberg, C. J., Keeler, E. B., & Ak, E. (1986). Chronic disease in a general adult population. *Western Journal of Medicine*, 145, 537–545.

Maina, G., Albert, U., Bogetto, F., Vaschetto, P., & Ravizza, L. (1999). Recent life events and obsessive-compulsive disorder (OCD): The role of pregnancy/delivery. *Psychiatry Research*, 89, 49–58.

Marazziti, D., Dell'Osso, L. G. A., Ciapparelli, A., Presta, S., Nasso, E. D., Pfanner, C., et al. (2001). Citalopram in refractory obsessive-compulsive disorder: An open study. *International Clinical Psychopharmacology*, 16, 215–219.

McDougle, C. J., Barr, L. C., Goodman, W. K., & Price, L. H. (1999). Possible role of neuropeptides in obsessive compulsive disorder. *Psychoneuroendocrinology*, 24, 1–4.

McEwen, B.S. (1998). Protective and damaging effects of stress mediators. *The New England Journal of Medicine*, 338, 171-179.

Metz, A. M., & Sichel, D. A. (1988). Postpartum panic disorder. *Journal of Clinical Psychiatry*, 49, 278–279.

Montgomery, S. A., Kasper, S., Stein, D. J., Bang Hedegaard, K., & Lemming, O. M. (2001). Citralopram 20 mg, 40 mg, and 60 mg are all effective and well tolerated compared with placebo in obsessive-compulsive disorder. *International Clinical Psychopharmacology*, 16, 75–86.

Montgomery, S. A., Montgomery, D. B., & Fineberg, N. (1990). Early response with clomipramine in obsessive-compulsive disorder: A placebo controlled study. *Prog Neuropsychopharmacological Biological Psychiatry*, 14, 719–727.

Pigott, T. A. (2002). Anxiety disorders. In A. H. Clayton (Ed.), *Women's mental health: A comprehensive textbook* (pp. 195–221). New York: The Guilford Press.

Sheehan, D. (1999). Current concepts in the treatment of panic disorder. *Journal of Clinical Psychiatry*, 60 (Suppl. 18), 16-21.

Sholomskas, D., Wickamaraine, P., Dogolo, L., O'Brien, D., Leaf, P., & Woods, S. (1993). Postpartum onset of panic disorder: A coincidental event? *Journal of Clinical Psychiatry*, 54, 476–480.

Sichel, D. A., Cohen, L. S., Dimmock, J. A., & Rosenbaum, J. F. (1993). Postpartum obsessive compulsive disorder: A case series. *Journal of Clinical Psychiatry*, 54, 156–159.

Sichel, D. A., Cohen, L. S., Rosenbaum, J. F., & Driscoll, J. W. (1993). Postpartum onset of obsessive-compulsive disorder. *Psychosomatics*, 34, 277–279.

Sichel, D. A., & Driscoll, J. W. (1999). *Women's moods: What every woman must know about the hormones, the brain, and emotional health*. New York: William Morrow Publishers.

Thoren, P., Asberg, M., Cronholm, B., Jornestedt, L., & Traskman, L. (1980). Clomipramine treatment in obsessive-compulsive disorder: I: A controlled clinical trial. *Archives in General Psychiatry*, 37, 1281–1285.

Tollefson, G. D., Rampey, A. H., Jr., Potvin, J. H., Jenike, M. A., Rush, A. J., Kominguez, R. A., et al. (1994). A multicenter investigation of fixed-dose fluoxetine in the treatment of obsessive-compulsive disorder. *Archives in General Psychiatry*, 51, 559–567.

Weaver, J. (1997). Childbirth: Preventing post-traumatic stress disorder. *Professional Care of Mother and Child*, 7, 2–3.

Williams, K. E., & Koran, L. M. (1997). Obsessive-compulsive disorder in pregnancy, the puerperium, and the premenstruum. *Journal of Clinical Psychiatry*, 58, 330–334.

Wisner, K. L., Peindl, K. S., & Hanusa, B. H. (1996). Effects of childbearing on the natural history of panic disorder with comorbid mood disorder. *Journal of Affective Disorders*, 41, 173–180.

Yonkers, K. A., & Kidner, C. L. (2002). Sex differences in anxiety disorders. In J. M. Herrera (Ed.), *Psychiatric illness in women* (pp. 5–30). Washington, DC: American Psychiatric Publishing.

Zohar, J., & Judge, R. (1996). Paroxetine versus clomipramine in the treatment of obsessive-compulsive disorder: OCD Paroxetine Study Investigators. *British Journal of Psychiatry*, 169, 468–474.

CHAPTER 8

POSTTRAUMATIC STRESS DISORDER SECONDARY TO BIRTH TRAUMA

Diagnostic Criteria for Posttraumatic Stress Disorder

A. The person has been exposed to a traumatic event in which both of the following were present:
1. The person experienced, witnessed, or was confronted with an event or events that involved actual or threatened death or serious injury or a threat to the physical integrity of self or others
2. The person's response involved intense fear, helplessness, or horror.

B. The traumatic event is persistently re-experienced in one (or more) of the following ways:
1. Recurrent and intrusive distressing recollections of the event, including images, thoughts, or perceptions
2. Recurrent distressing dreams of the event
3. Acting or feeling as if the traumatic event were recurring (includes a sense of reliving the experience, illusions, hallucinations, and dissociative flashback episodes, including those that occur on awakening or when intoxicated)
4. Intense psychologic distress at exposure to internal or external cues that symbolize or resemble an aspect of the traumatic event

  5. Physiologic reactivity on exposure to internal or external cues that symbolize or resemble an aspect of the traumatic event

C. Persistent avoidance of stimuli associated with the trauma and numbing of general responsiveness (not present before the trauma), as indicated by three (or more) of the following:

  1. Efforts to avoid thoughts, feelings, or conversations associated with the trauma

  2. Efforts to avoid activities, places, or people that arouse recollections of the trauma

  3. Inability to recall an important aspect of the trauma

  4. Markedly diminished interest or participation in significant activities

  5. Feeling of detachment or estrangement from others

  6. Restricted range of affect (e.g., unable to have loving feelings)

  7. Sense of a foreshortened future (e.g., does not expect to have a career, marriage, children, or a normal life span)

D. Persistent symptoms of increased arousal (not present before the trauma), as indicated by two (or more) of the following:

  1. Difficulty falling or staying asleep

  2. Irritability or outbursts of anger

  3. Difficulty concentrating

  4. Hypervigilance

  5. Exaggerated startle response

E. Duration of the disturbance (symptoms in Criteria B, C, and D) is more than 1 month.

F. The disturbance causes clinically significant distress or impairment in social, occupational, or other important areas of functioning.

Specify if:

  Acute: If duration of symptoms is less than 3 months

  Chronic: If duration of symptoms is 3 months or more

Specify if: With delayed onset if onset is 6 months after the stressor (American Psychiatric Association, 2000, pp. 467–468)

Reprinted with permission from the *Diagnostic and Statistical Manual of Mental Disorders.* Copyright 2000, American Psychiatric Association.

Posttraumatic stress disorder (PTSD) caused by childbirth is the focus of this chapter. First, a general overview of the prevalence of PTSD after childbirth is presented. After a description of mothers' experiences of traumatic births, the aftermath of birth trauma, PTSD, is addressed. Treatment and a case study are included in this chapter.

PTSD Caused by Childbirth

In 1980, PTSD was first included in the *Diagnostic and Statistical Manual of Mental Disorders* (DSM-III) (American Psychiatric Association, 1980). Vietnam War veterans were the initial persons identified as having PTSD. In the DSM-III, one of the criteria required for the diagnosis of PTSD was an event that was considered beyond the range of usual human experience. The DSM-IV provided a broadened view of what constituted an extreme traumatic stressor to include "direct personal experience of an event that involves actual or threatened death or serious injury, or a threat to the physical integrity of self or others" (American Psychological Association, 1994, p. 424). The person's response is one of extreme fear, helplessness, or horror. Although childbirth is not specifically classified as an example of an extremely traumatic stressor, it certainly can qualify as a traumatic event (Beck, 2004a).

The reported prevalence of diagnosed PTSD caused by childbirth ranges from 1.5% (Ayers & Pickering, 2001) to 6% (Menage, 1993). Wijma, Soderquist, and Wijma (1997) examined the prevalence of PTSD caused by childbirth in Sweden using the Traumatic Event Scale (Wijma et al.). Twenty-eight of 1,640 women (1.7%) met the criteria for PTSD. Factors related to the women's experience of PTSD after childbirth included a history of psychiatric counseling, a negative cognitive appraisal of the past delivery, nulliparity, and negative contact with the delivery staff.

Creedy, Shochet, and Horsfall (2000) identified a 5.6% prevalence of PTSD caused by childbirth (28 of 99 women) in Australia. Diagnosis was based on the Posttraumatic Symptoms Interview (Foa, Riggs, Dancu, & Rothbaum, 1993), which was conducted at 4 to 6 weeks postpartum. Stressful birth events included extreme pain, a mother's fear for her own life or for her infant's life, and a perception of a real or actual lack of obstetric care. Two variables were associated significantly with acute trauma symptoms: a high degree of obstetric intervention and dissatisfaction with the care received during labor and delivery.

Using the Posttraumatic Symptoms Interview (Foa et al., 1993), Ayers and Pickering (2001) measured the prevalence of PTSD at 6 weeks and 6 months postpartum. Of a sample of 218 mothers in the United Kingdom, 2.8% fulfilled criteria for PTSD at 6 weeks postpartum, and this number decreased to 1.5% at 6 months postpartum.

Menage (1993) identified a prevalence rate for PTSD caused by childbirth of 6% in the United Kingdom. The PTSD Interview of the Veterans Administration Medical Center in Minnesota (Watson, Juba, Manifold, Kucala, & Anderson, 1991) was used to diagnose PTSD. Thirty of 500 mothers satisfied the DSM-III criteria for PTSD.

The only study to date conducted in the United States identified a prevalence rate of 1.9% (Soet, Brack, & Dilorio, 2003). Of a sample of 103, two women were diagnosed with PTSD after childbirth at 4 weeks postpartum. The woman's experience of birth trauma was measured using the Traumatic Event Scale (Wijma et al., 1997). Significant predictors of birth trauma included cesarean delivery, medical intervention, long and painful labor, feelings of powerlessness, inadequate information, a negative interaction with medical personnel, and differences between expectations and the actual event of childbirth.

In other studies, posttraumatic stress symptoms were examined, but a formal diagnosis of PTSD was not made. In Sweden, Ryding, Wijma, and Wijma (1998) compared the psychologic impact of emergency cesarean birth (N = 71) with elective cesarean birth (N = 70), instrumental (N = 89), and normal vaginal delivery (N = 96). Posttraumatic stress symptoms were measured using the Impact of Events Scale (Horowitz, Wilner, & Alvarez, 1979) 4 weeks after delivery. Women who had an emergency cesarean delivery reported significantly more posttraumatic stress symptoms than the elective cesarean and normal spontaneous delivery women but not when compared with the mothers who had instrumental vaginal deliveries. In this study, 29 women (55%) reported experiencing intense fear of death or injury to themselves or to their baby during birth, which fulfilled the stressor criterion of DSM-IV. The most common fear was focused on concerns that the baby would die or be injured. The women who feared for their own lives had experienced a painful labor. The results indicated that 8% of the mothers were angry because they felt that the delivery staff had treated them very badly. These women felt violated and helpless during the care provided by the delivery staff.

Lyons (1998) also measured posttraumatic stress symptoms 4 weeks after delivery using the Impact of Events Scale (Horowitz et al., 1979) with 42 primiparas in the United Kingdom. Higher posttraumatic stress symptoms were significantly related to the feeling of not being in control during delivery, being induced, and having an epidural.

Czarnocka and Slade (2000) investigated the prevalence and potential predictors of posttraumatic stress symptoms with a sample of 246 women in the United Kingdom. At 6 weeks postpartum, the mothers completed the Posttraumatic Stress Disorder Questionnaire and Interview (Watson et al., 1991). Three percent of the sample (n = 8) reported symptoms on the Posttraumatic Stress Disorder Questionnaire indicating clinically significant levels of the three posttraumatic stress dimensions: intrusions, avoidance, and hyperarousal. Regression analysis indicated the following significant predictors of posttraumatic stress symptoms related to childbirth: low levels of perceived support from labor and delivery staff and partner and low perceived control during labor.

In Canada, posttraumatic stress was examined in 200 mothers 8 to 10 weeks after delivery (Cohen, Ansara, Schei, Stuckless, & Stewart, 2004). Women were interviewed by telephone with the Davidson Trauma Scale (DTS) (Davidson, Book, Colket, & Tupler, 1977). The DTS is a 17-item scale that measures the 17 DSM-IV symptoms of PTSD. Postpartum stress was categorized as high postpartum stress (answered "yes" to three or more items) or low postpartum stress (answered "yes" to zero to two items). Logistic regression analysis indicated that significant risk factors of high postpartum stress were experiencing two or more maternal complications after labor and delivery, depression during pregnancy, being born in Canada, higher household income, and a large number of lifetime traumatic events. Women who scored high on the EPDS were also likely to score high on the DTS.

Posttraumatic stress symptoms have been found at a significantly higher level in mothers of high-risk infants (Callahan & Hynan, 2002; DeMier, Hynan, Harris, & Manniello, 1996) than in mothers of healthy, full-term infants. Posttraumatic stress symptoms in mothers of premature infants were assessed by Holditch-Davis, Bartlett, Blickman, and Miles (2003) using a semistructured interview with 30 mothers at 6 months after delivery. The interviews were analyzed for three PTSD symptoms: re-experiencing, avoidance, and increased arousal. Twenty-four of the 30 mothers reported avoiding thinking about aspects of the birth/neonatal intensive care unit (NICU) and re-experiencing the preterm birth of their infant through intrusive thoughts. Twenty-six women described increased arousal that focused on overprotecting their infant as a type of hypervigilance. Women reported difficulty sleeping and generalized anxiety, and also experienced persistent fears that their child might die or become ill again.

In her grounded theory study, Allen (1998) investigated the processes that happened during traumatic childbirth, the mediating variables in the development of PTSD symptoms, and the impact on postpartum adaptation. Twenty mothers were interviewed 10 months after delivery. The Revised Impact of Events Scale (Horowitz et al., 1979) was used to assess PTSD symptoms. Six women reported scores above the cutoff point, indicating clinically significant levels of PTSD symptoms after childbirth. Their distress included panic and tearfulness caused by thoughts of the trauma, anger directed at labor and delivery staff and their partners, decreased closeness in their relationships with their partners, emotional detachment from the baby, less patience with their other children, and fear of future pregnancy.

Grounded theory analysis indicated that the core category related to a traumatic birth experience was the women's feelings of not being in control of events of their own behavior. Causal factors resulting in the perception of a traumatic birth were the belief that the infant would be harmed, past experiences in labor, and pain during labor. The women tried to gain control by seeking reassurance and knowledge provided by staff and partners.

Birth Trauma

What are the essential elements of a birth that could be so traumatic that it would lead to PTSD? I investigated this question in a phenomenologic study with 40 mothers who had experienced birth trauma (Beck, 2004a).

The study results clearly show that birth trauma is in the eye of the beholder. The birth traumas identified by the women in the sample are presented in Table 8.1. The concept of birth trauma involves traumatic experiences that may occur during any phase of childbearing. During any phase, the trauma may be classified as a negative outcome, including a stillbirth, an obstetric complication (e.g., an emergency cesarean), or psychologic distress (fear of an epidural). The following four themes were revealed in my study that describe the essence of birth trauma:

"Theme 1: To care for me: Was that too much to ask?

"I am amazed that 3.5 hours in the labor and delivery room could cause such utter destruction in my life. It truly was like being the victim of a violent crime or rape."

What could have happened to this woman and others to turn the delivery process into a rape scene? A perceived lack of caring approach during such a vulnerable time was one of the core components in this scenario for a traumatic birth. The mothers reported that feeling abandoned and alone, feeling stripped of their dignity, a lack of interest in them as unique persons, and a lack of support and reassurance all contributed to their birth trauma. One mother said she *"felt betrayed by a system that is supposedly there to care for me."*

The women who participated in this study reported that their expectations for their labor and delivery care were shattered. One mother painfully stated this:

> *The labor care has hurt deep in my soul, and I have no words to describe the hurt. I was treated like nothing, just someone to get data from. The nurse took my pulse, temperature, blood pressure, and weight without talking to me as a person. She then asked about teeth, colds, and smoking without acknowledging me as a person. She left me, tears rolling down my face.*

A multipara who had an induced labor said this:

> *I felt like just a vessel into which you poured hormones hoping for the quick release of another baby.*

The adjectives used by the mothers in this study to describe the care they had received during the delivery process included "mechanical," "arrogant," "cold," "technical," and "lack of empathy." For example, within

---

Table 8.1   LIST OF BIRTH TRAUMAS

- Stillbirth/infant death
- Emergency cesarean delivery/fetal distress
- Cardiac arrest
- Inadequate medical care
- Fear of epidural
- Congenital anomalies
- Inadequate pain relief
- Postpartum hemorrhage/manual removal of placenta
- Forceps/vacuum extraction/skull fracture
- Severe toxemia
- Premature birth
- Separation from infant in NICU
- Prolonged, painful labor
- Rapid delivery
- Degrading experience

Reprinted with permission from Beck, Birth trauma: In the eye of the beholder. *Nursing Research*, 53, p. 32, 2004a.

24 hours of giving birth, one mother had to say goodbye forever to her beloved newborn daughter. As her baby was dying in the NICU, her husband took lots of photos until the film ran out. She and her husband asked for more film and ignored the disapproving looks of the staff members. They wondered, *"Was this too much to ask for—for us, it was our only opportunity to do this before our daughter died."*

The mothers reported that being stripped of their dignity also played a part in their birth trauma. As one young Puerto Rican mother recounted,

> *They had me in all kinds of positions (including all fours) to hear the heartbeat with the stethoscope, and about 20 students came in the room without my permission. All I heard them saying was that I was now 7.5 dilated. By the way, while I was on all fours, I was trying to cover my bottom by holding the gown. So, I felt raped, and my dignity was taken from me.*

During the delivery process, some women were shaken to the core by feeling abandoned and alone:

> *"I had a major bleed and started shaking involuntarily all over. Even my jaw shook, and I couldn't stop. I heard the specialist say he was having trouble stopping the bleeding. I was very frightened, and then it hit me. I might not make it! I can still recall the sick dread of real fear. I needed urgent reassurance, but none was offered."*

Theme 2: To communicate with me: Why was this neglected?

At times, the mothers perceived that the labor and delivery staff failed to communicate with their patients. During a traumatic birth, women often felt invisible. Clinicians spoke to each other as if the woman was not present. One woman who was having her first baby recalled:

> *After an hour of trying to deliver the baby with a vacuum extractor, the obstetrician said it that was too late for an emergency cesarean. The baby was truly stuck. By now the doctors are acting like I'm not there. The attending physician was saying, "We may have lost this bloody baby." The hospital staff discussed my baby's possible death in front of me and argued in front of me just as if I weren't there.*

The following segment of a mother's story dramatically illustrates how someone merely communicating with her and explaining what was happening could have prevented her birth trauma:

> The doctor turned on this machine that sounded like a swimming
> pool pump. He proceeded and hurriedly showed me the piece that
> was to be inserted into me. It was chrome metal and extremely
> large in circumference. Next thing he begins to pull on this hose,
> which was the extension of the suction. He gritted his teeth and
> pulled. I felt sick. On the other end of the machine was our baby's
> head. He used every ounce of his male strength to pull the baby
> out. I was horrified. I started to imagine how any minute a head
> would come out, ripped off its body. I was really in shock. He had
> his foot up on the bed, using it as leverage to pull. All of a
> sudden, the loud sucking machine made an even louder noise,
> and it broke suction. The doctor fell back and nearly landed on
> his bum. Blood came spurting out of me, all over him. That was it
> for me. I thought he'd ripped the head off. He then swore and
> said hurriedly, "Get the forceps." I can still remember the feeling
> of him ripping the baby out of me. It was the most awful, unnatu-
> ral, devastating feeling ever. Well, finally, out came this baby.
> I was, by this stage, still stuck in my own private horror movie,
> visualizing my baby being born dead with half of its head
> missing. The pediatrician was standing beside the doctor, and I
> assumed that he would take the dead baby away. But, much to
> my horror and surprise, the doctor pulled out this blood red baby,
> and threw it onto my tummy. I screamed, "Get him off me!"
> I cried my eyes out!

Clinicians also at times failed to communicate among themselves, which influenced the women's perceptions of their deliveries as traumatic. For example, labor was induced for one woman who had experienced a previous serious vasovagal reaction before pregnancy, and it came time for her to receive an epidural. She was terrified because the midwife did not tell the anesthetist about her history. As this mother shared,

> I remember my husband trying to tell the anesthetist that I was
> fearful of a vasovagal attack. The midwife should have been doing
> that. My husband kept saying, "My wife, my wife." He could not
> remember what to say. I was terrified for my life. My soul was in
> agony because the medical people did not know the situation. I was
> terrified to the core of my being. I called out, "I'm scared. I'm
> scared." Not scared of the needle, scared for my life.

Theme 3: To provide safe care: You betrayed my trust and I felt powerless.

Women began their labors confident that the delivery staff would provide safe care. The women entrusted their lives and those of their unborn babies into the hands of these clinicians. At times, women perceived that they received unsafe care, which ignited terror in them as they feared for their own safety and that of their infants but felt powerless to rectify the dangerous situation. As one mother vehemently recounted:

> I remember believing that the labor and delivery team would know what was right and would be there should things go wrong. That was my first mistake. They didn't, and they weren't! I strongly believe my PTSD was caused by feelings of powerlessness and loss of control of what people did to my body.

One brief scenario vividly illustrates this third theme. Shortly before becoming pregnant the second time, one mother had surgery to repair a hiatal hernia. During this pregnancy, gestational diabetes developed, and at 28 weeks, a scan detected a mass in the brain of her fetus. Her desired birth plan was to have caesarean delivery to save her baby the distress of a vaginal birth. The doctor "pressured" her into the trial of labor because her first delivery had been so straightforward and rapid. The doctor assures her that if she got into difficulties she could "easily convert to cesarean." As this mother explained,

> I went into the delivery room assured that my baby and I would be in safe hands. I got into difficulties at 9 p.m. with severe abdominal pain and felt that something was terribly wrong. I was in what I describe as "white pain," a terrible ripping pain. I told the staff something was wrong and I begged for caesarean. I was pushing for hours to no avail, flat on my back, numb from the waist down and feeling that my vague pushes were killing my unborn daughter. I started to die inside. The whole of my genital area was swollen to resemble a baboon. My daughter was posterior, brow presenting, and I continued in second stage labor actively pushing for over 6 hours. My daughter was distressed and her heartbeat kept disappearing. An episiotomy was cut without so much as eye contact with me. My daughter was born flat, resuscitated with apgars of 2 and 6, and taken to the NICU. After being stitched up, I went to see my baby, and I didn't recognize her, felt no bond—nothing. She wasn't my baby; my baby had died. In my mind, my efforts to

give birth had killed her. After delivery, I was incontinent. The
familiar stomach pain returned. My hiatus hernia repair had now
failed. I later had repair surgery to reattach a part of my labia
majora. I had an anal sphincter repair, and my pelvic floor was re-
fashioned at the same time. I'm waiting for repeat hiatus hernia
repair, and I am still going to physiotherapy to improve the inconti-
nence. During labor, I had expected pain, and I had expected a
powerful experience. I expected that, if necessary, medical staff
would intervene to keep us safe. Why didn't anyone use their pro-
fessional judgment? That was what I expected from them. I have
posttraumatic stress disorder.

Theme 4: The end justifies the means: At whose expense? At what price?
Mothers believed that the bottom line in considering a delivery a successful experience was the outcome of the baby. If the baby was born alive
with good Apgar scores, that was what mattered to the labor and delivery
staff and even to the mother's family and friends. The safe arrival of a live,
healthy infant symbolized the achievement of clinical efficiency and professional and fiscal goals. Mothers perceived that their traumatic deliveries were glossed over and pushed into the background as the healthy
newborn took center stage. Why put a damper on this celebration by
focusing on mother's traumatic experience giving birth?

One woman had been hospitalized with chronic sciatica 20 years earlier
when she was 18 years old. She received an epidural steroid injection for
treatment. As the woman recalled,

> *The needle hit a nerve in my back and created a frightful situation*
> *where I could not move. I had such a horrible sensation that I vowed*
> *on the spot never, ever to have another epidural.*

Submitting to her most dreaded epidural and saying goodbye to her
dreams of a vaginal delivery, this woman experienced an out-of-body experience as she lay on the delivery table hemorrhaging. She wrote,

> *I would have done anything to have this baby and did everything,*
> *even stuff I didn't want to. All that I get told when dealing with the*
> *residual emotional effects is, "You should be happy with the outcome."*

After an hour of pushing, one primipara was offered forceps. The
epidural was topped up but not given enough time to work properly, nor
was it checked. The mother felt the cut, the forceps going in, and her body

tearing as the doctor pulled the baby out. She screamed loud and long. She shared that she

> *Was congratulated for how "quickly and easily" the baby came out and that he scored a perfect 10! The worst thing was that nobody acknowledged that I had a bad time. Everyone was so pleased that it had gone so well! I felt as if I had been raped!*

Women who perceived that they had experienced traumatic births viewed the site of their labor and delivery as a battlefield. Although engaged in the battle, their protective layers were stripped away, leaving them exposed to the onslaught of birth trauma. Stripped from these women were their individuality, dignity, control, communication, caring, trust, and support and reassurance."

Reprinted with permission from Beck, Birth trauma: In the eye of the beholder. *Nursing Research,* 54, pp. 32-34 2004a.

PTSD Caused by Childbirth: The Aftermath

After completing the study on birth trauma, I continued to conduct research and now turned my attention to investigating the aftermath of traumatic births. I next conducted a phenomenologic study with 38 women who had experienced PTSD caused by birth trauma (Beck, 2004b). The following five themes emerged from the mothers' stories of their experiences of PTSD after childbirth (Table 8.2).

Theme 1: Going to the movies: Please don't make me go!
Mothers suffering from PTSD were bombarded not only during the day with flashbacks reliving their traumatic births but also during the night with terrifying nightmares. Women repeatedly used the image of a video on automatic replay or loop tracks imprinted in their brains to describe how uncontrollable the distressing memories or "movies" of their traumatic childbirths were to them.

A primipara who had a failed vacuum extraction followed by a forceps delivery and a fourth degree tear provided an illustration of these loop tracks that left her feeling like she was "faking it" and stuck in the past, unable to enjoy the present with her infant:

I lived in two worlds, the videotape of the birth and the "real" world. The videotape felt more real. I lived in my own bubble, not quite connecting with anyone. I could hear and communicate but experienced interaction with others as a spectator. The "videotape" ran constantly for 4 months.

Another mother who also had a failed vacuum extraction followed by a forceps delivery desperately wanted to get out of this nightmare she was starring in. As she explained, "I had nightmares of my delivery doctor as a rapist, coming knocking on my door. I also believed when my son was born that the doctor had ripped his head off. These two images were what affected my existence."

Table 8.2   FIVE ESSENTIAL THEMES OF PTSD CAUSED BY CHILDBIRTH

THEME NUMBER		THEME
1		Going to the movies: Please don't make me go!
2		A shadow of myself: Too numb to try and change
3		Seeking to have questions answered and wanting to talk, talk, talk
4		The dangerous trio of anger, anxiety, and depression: Spiraling downward
5		Isolation from the world of motherhood: Dreams shattered

Adapted and reprinted with permission from Beck, Posttraumatic stress disorder due to childbirth: The aftermath. *Nursing Research*, 53, p. 220, 2004b.

One woman who had been refused an epidural and had an "agonizing forceps delivery" suffered from "extraordinarily realistic nightmares." She shared, "*Like Lady MacBeth, I became terrified of sleeping! I would go without sleep for about 72 to 96 hours. I always knew I'd have to fight the nightmares again. I was scared that this time I wouldn't have the strength to fight it—that it would succeed in destroying me.*"

Flashbacks and nightmares of the traumatic births affected not only mothers' relationships with their children but also with their husbands. One multipara who had experienced a high level of medical intervention during the delivery shared this: "*After about 6 months my husband and I still hadn't had sex since before the birth. When we began to try, I had flashbacks to the birth. At the moment of penetration, I would have a flashback to the instant when my body was pulled down the operating table during one of the failed forceps attempts.*"

Theme 2: A shadow of myself: Too numb to try and change.

Traumatized by their birth experience, mothers suffering from PTSD considered themselves only as a shadow of their former selves. This numbing of self, and for some women actually dissociating, can began immediately after delivery. One woman who had an emergency cesarean and postpartum hemorrhage vividly described that after delivery she was "*put in a room with two other mothers. I had a drip and a catheter, and I was silent. I felt completely numb. I did what was required and I felt that my head was floating way above my body. I struggled to bring it back onto my shoulders. I still feel dissociated like this sometimes.*"

Another mother who had hemorrhaged on the delivery table recalled when she was wheeled out to the recovery room. "*My parents were there, as was my sister. I did not cry or smile. I watched them looking happy. I was completely numb and could not remember any emotional context to do with my delivery day. The midwife pointed my baby out to me in the nursery as I was wheeled by. He was so big. I felt no recognition. I felt nothing.*"

Once home, these feelings of numbness and detachment continued. One primipara who had a terrifying experience with an epidural shared, "*I'd wake up numb, unable to feel a thing. I'd drag myself through the day. I am having the hardest time trying to overcome this feeling of being dead.*" Another woman poignantly described feeling as though her soul had left her and she was now only an empty shell. "*Mechanically, I'd go through the motions of being a good mother. Inside, I felt nothing. If the emotion did start to leak, I quickly suppressed it. I'd smack myself on the hand and put my 'robot suit' back on.*"

Theme 3: Seeking to have questions answered and wanting to talk, talk, talk.

Mothers suffering from PTSD had an intense need to know the details of their traumatic births and to get answers to their questions. These women obsessed over trying to understand what had happened and why it had happened. This obsession took on many different forms. For some women, it entailed making repeated appointments with the physicians or midwives who had delivered their infants to have their questions answered and to go over their hospital records. Reading obstetrical text-books was the way other women spent their free time when they were not caring for their infants.

Revisiting the delivery room/OB theater became necessary for some women, even as long as a year after birth. One multipara whose request for pain medications during labor had been denied, shared this: "*At the first birthday of my little daughter, I had a horrible recurrence of the* PTSD. *I insisted that the hospital let me visit the delivery room and threatened them with a lawsuit if they didn't grant my request.*"

Women experiencing PTSD revealed that they wanted to talk, talk, talk about their traumatic births, but they discovered quite quickly that health care providers and family members became tired of listening. After her traumatic delivery, a mother of multiples revealed that "I was so devastated at people's lack of empathy. I told myself what a bad person I was for needing to talk. I felt like the Ancient Mariner doomed to forever be plucking at people's sleeves and trying to tell them my story, which they didn't want to hear."

Eventually, some women stopped discussing their traumatic births, which became detrimental to their mental health. As one woman explained, "*I didn't communicate with anyone anymore. The room I was in became my cave. I was consumed by my birth demon.*" Their unasked, unanswered questions "gnawed away" at them.

One mother of multiples who had an emergency cesarean poignantly tried to express in words what happened,

> *Not only does* PTSD *isolate me from the outside world, it isolates me even from those I love. How do I explain the sort of blind terror that overtakes me without warning and without obvious logical cause? And what of my family and friends? They don't know how I feel. They don't know what to say. They cannot make it better, so they end up feeling useless. That's the real problem with* PTSD.

It separates people at the time when love and understanding are most needed. It's like an invisible wall around the sufferer.

After repeated unsuccessful attempts at trying to get satisfactory answers about their traumatic births or at least an apology from their health care providers and the hospital, some women took their quest to a higher level. Examples of this next step included taking their cause to the Health and Disability Commissioner, filing an accident compensation claim, and submitting a formal complaint to the state medical board. When, for instance, the state medical board sided with the physicians, women stated that they were "retraumatized." As one woman who had experienced an emergency cesarean delivery painfully shared, *"The emotional pain of this secondary wounding was worse than the actual physical pain of labor."*

Theme 4: The dangerous trio of anger, anxiety, and depression: Spiraling downward.

This trio of distressing emotions permeated the daily lives of mothers suffering from PTSD. Women experienced these emotions on a heightened level. Anger was rage. Anxiety turned into panic attacks, and depression left many suicidal. Anger was directed in multiple directions. Its stinging tentacles lashed out at health care providers, family members, and self. Marital relationships were at times strained to the limit. As one mother whose firstborn infant had died explained, *"To live daily with the fact that you were like a time bomb ready to go off was dreadful. As time went on, I knew I was personally 'too hot to handle' and not nice to be with, as invariably you could not help but have some of your inner state ooze or jump out at those who did come close."*

Another woman revealed that *"the powerful seething anger would overwhelm me without warning. To manage it, I would go still and quiet, then eventually 'come to,' realizing that one or all of the children were crying and I had no idea for how long."*

Mothers experiencing PTSD also turned their anger inward at times toward themselves. A mother who had given birth to twins shared that she was so full of anger at herself. *"How could I have let this happen? Why did I trust the doctors? How could I have been so stupid?"*

Women were angry with the labor and delivery staff who they perceived betrayed their trust and let them down. This anger was not a fleeting emotion. A mother whose infant sustained a skull fracture from a vacuum extraction 3 years earlier shared that she still sometimes "relives" the traumatic birth and is still really angry and mistrustful of doctors

Anxiety also plagued women suffering from PTSD caused by birth trauma. For some mothers, the anxiety began on the delivery table. As a woman who had experienced "excruciating" pain once her membranes had been artificially ruptured shared, "I *had intense pains in my chest from the first moment after the birth that have been extremely difficult to get rid of. They turned into anxiety.*" After her traumatic birth, one primipara became extremely anxious regarding intercourse, causing her to have a nonintimate relationship for most of the next 9 years. One mother was so anxious that she made sores in her scalp and face. Women who had never experienced panic attacks before their birth trauma began to be plagued by them. One mother whose infant had received cuts and bruises due to a forceps delivery experienced panic attacks whenever she went to a hospital or doctor's office.

Depression at times became severe enough to lead some mothers to contemplate ending their own lives. A mother of multiples shared, "*I wanted to kill myself. My life was a mess. Death seemed like a wonderful idea. I'd fight with myself while driving, 'put your foot on the brake, the light's red. No, don't put your foot on the brake,' and so it went on.*"

Theme 5: Isolation from the world of motherhood: Dreams shattered.

The tightening grip of PTSD after childbirth choked off three lifelines to the world of motherhood: (1) the woman's infant, (2) the supporting circle of other mothers, and (3) hopes for any additional children. Concentrating first on the present, some women shared that much to their dismay their PTSD distanced them from their infants. As one mother who had an unplanned cesarean delivery painfully remembered, "*At night I tried to connect/acknowledge in my heart that this was my son, and I cried. I knew that there were great layers of trauma around my heart. I wanted to feel motherhood. I wanted to experience and embrace it. Why was I chained up in the vice-like grip of this pain? This was my Gethsemane—my agony in the garden.*"

The walls that the birth trauma erected between mother and infant do not appear to be temporary for some mothers. As a multipara who survived a severe postpartum hemorrhage 3 years earlier painfully shared, her PTSD still holds a destructive grip on her relationship with her son.

> *My child turned 3 years old a few weeks ago. I suppose the pain was not so acute this time. I actually made him a birthday cake and was grateful that I could go to work and not think about the significance of the day. The pain was less, but it was replaced by a numbness that still worries me. I hope that as time passes I can forge some kind of real closeness with this child. I am still unable to tell him I love*

him, but I can now hold him and have times when I am proud of
him. I have come a long, long way.

PTSD also resulted in women isolating themselves from other mothers and babies. Mothers with PTSD could not tolerate or cope being with other women who had not experienced traumatic births. One mother would ask the nurse to schedule her baby's well-child checkups 15 minutes before the clinic opened so that she would not have to see or meet other mothers.

To have more children or not? What a heart-wrenching decision this was for mothers suffering from PTSD. For some women, the only choice for them was to have a tubal ligation, and one woman asked her husband to have a vasectomy. The following passage poignantly illustrates this: "*I couldn't envision EVER having another baby. There was no way I could expose myself again to that degree of vulnerability and abandonment. My little girl was the most precious thing in my life, but events that occurred at her birth mean that I will not be having anymore children. I had a tubal ligation, and I grieved for the babies I thought I wouldn't have.*"

For other women, even though they were terrified of going through another childbirth, they opted to have another child. Proactive planning and an "iron clad" birth plan helped to prepare the PTSD mothers for a second childbirth. Throughout her second pregnancy, one mother kept a diary as she struggled with her PTSD. One entry from her diary vividly illustrates how vulnerable and fragile these women are as the bravely face another childbirth. "*While I am trying to put my PTSD behind me, I am having to prepare for the birth of my second child. My reality is that I am scared—heart and womb. I need special care. My heart is fragile, and I am trying to protect it.*" In her diary, this mother who had an emergency cesarean with her first delivery kept a list of questions she was going to ask different midwives to help her choose a midwife she felt she could trust.

A sampling of these questions from her diary includes the following:

> *Why are you a midwife? How would you describe your approach*
> *to women in labor? What is the difference between being*
> *delivered and giving birth? What do you do when a woman in*
> *labor starts saying "I'm scared" as you commence a procedure?*"

Reprinted with permission from Beck, Posttraumatic stress disorder due to childbirth: The aftermath. *Nursing Research, 53,* pp. 219–222, 2004b.

Clinical Implications Based on Cheryl's Research

Based on Cheryl's birth trauma/PTSD caused by childbirth (Beck, 2004a, 2004b), she has derived the following implications for clinical practice:

- Be alert to the predictors of PTSD after childbirth, such as a high level of obstetric intervention during labor and delivery.
- Be vigilant in recognizing symptoms of PTSD or previous trauma during the prenatal, intrapartum, and postpartum periods, such as extreme fear or lack of trust of clinicians, dissociation, intense need to control labor, and flashbacks (Crompton, 1996; Kennedy & MacDonald, 2002).
- Be alert that labor and delivery can retraumatize mothers who have experienced previous trauma.
- Provide debriefing sessions for mothers who perceive their labor and delivery as traumatic.
- Provide mothers with the website of Trauma and Birth Stress, which is composed of other women who have experienced birth trauma/PTSD caused by childbirth (www.tabs.org.nz).
- Be cognizant of the devastating effects of PTSD not only on the mother but also on her relationship with her infant.
- Take a careful history from each woman at her admission to labor and delivery regarding any specific fears that she may have about giving birth and about whether previous deliveries were perceived as traumatic.
- Treat each woman during labor and delivery as though she were a survivor of previous trauma (Church & Scanlan, 2002).

Treatment

The treatment of PTSD secondary to birth trauma may include psychotherapy, psychopharmacology, and eye movement desensitization and reprocessing (EMDR). As we have discussed frequently in this book, the relationship is critical to the healing process. The woman suffering from PTSD may present with what looks like a generalized anxiety disorder until you begin to uncover the experiences that led to the trauma. It is difficult for a woman to disclose personal feelings in a culture that has been supporting the fact that she is alive and her baby is alive. She feels that she should just be happy with that. However, as she keeps suppressing her feelings and responses to the birth trauma, her symptoms can exacerbate and lead to severe anxiety disorder, depression, and even suicidal ideation and intent. Sensitive, comprehensive assessment is critical to uncover and allow her voice to be heard. After the story has been told, validated, and honored, in my opinion (Jeanne), the treatment has begun.

Based on my clinical practice, psychopharmacology is often necessary immediately so that the biological symptoms of insomnia, anxiety, irritation, fear, and potential phobias can be quieted and the woman can feel a bit more in control. Education and anticipatory guidance regarding medications are critical, as one wants to avoid the potential retraumatization that may occur with side effects of medications if not judiciously chosen.

PTSD is a form of a subcategory of anxiety disorder, and many of the biological treatment strategies are the same. The SSRI antidepressants constitute first-line pharmacotherapy for PTSD (Davidson & Connor, 1999; Marshall & Pierce, 2000; Rothbaum, Ninan, & Thomas, 1996). TCAs and MAOIs are also effective and should be considered for patients with PTSD who fail to respond to SSRI treatment (Davidson & Connor, 1999). The SSRI antidepressants appear to have a broad spectrum of activity in the treatment of the symptoms of PTSD. The treatment should be initiated at a relatively low dose and maintained for at least 12 months before discontinuing (Pigott, 2002). Many common symptoms—anxiety, insomnia, an exaggerated startle response, intrusive trauma-related recollections, feelings of emotional numbing, and avoidance behaviors—have been reported to improve with SSRI treatment (Davidson & Connor, 1999). However, the use of antianxiety agents (i.e., benzodiazepines) is generally considered an adjunct to the treatment with antidepressant agents, as they can decrease the arousal states and treat the insomnia (Hendrick & Gitlin, 2004).

Interestingly, if one considers biological interactions, alterations in the hypothalamic–pituitary–adrenal axis have been implicated in PTSD. In women, there are obvious fluctuations in estrogen and progesterone, with dramatic drops in these hormones during the acute postpartum phase (Chrousos, Torpy, & Gold, 1998). This biochemical implication may indeed have a significant impact on the reactions and responses of women to traumatic birth experiences. Unfortunately, as we have seen, very little systematic research or information is available pertaining to these specific endocrine effects in women and their biology.

Supportive psychotherapy, in conjunction with the pharmacotherapy, is imperative during the early stages of treatment in that the woman has a place to establish trust and feel secure in disclosing her story. Also, there is the goal of providing a healing experience in the relationship. I (Jeanne) have found that after the symptoms have abated and the woman feels more in control that cognitive–behavioral strategies are helpful. Interestingly, in my experience as a clinician in working with women with PTSD secondary to birth trauma, the women have gone on to have more children. However, new obstetrical providers were secured. Locations of birth were changed, and there was significant time spent on relationship development and verbal contract development with providers regarding the woman's experiences and potential needs. For some women, we have had to located a provider who would agree to an elective cesarean birth, as that would eliminate the trauma of another birth experience. For other women, a vaginal birth experience was important to their healing trajectory. Again, the individuality of the woman must be a major factor in the care plan development and implementation.

Case Study

Kesha called on the phone. Her primary care provider had given her my name and phone number. "I don't know what is wrong with me. I am a nervous wreck. I feel nauseous all of the time and have episodes of diarrhea. I am having nightmares, and it feels like panic attacks. He did some tests, but everything is normal. He said to call you—that you might be able to help me."

When Kesha comes to my office, she is an attractive woman, is neatly dressed, and appears to be a bit nervous, as she kept playing with her car keys. I asked her to fill out the admission forms and got her a glass of water; then we began the assessment process. Initially, I let Kesha tell me her story to find out "how her brain got here" (Sichel & Driscoll, 1999). Kesha described that for the past few months she has been having bad dreams, major anxiety attacks, and just feeling scared all the time. She had a baby 1 year ago and felt that she did fine after the baby was born. She is unsure what is going on now. Using the Earthquake Assessment, I proceeded to collect the data regarding her genetic, hormonal, and stress response history.

Kesha is 30 years old and the first child with two siblings. Her parents are alive and well and live in another state. Currently, she lives with her boyfriend and father of her baby, Sam. "We are getting married in 6 months." She denies any mood or anxiety disorders in her parents, although she does state that "my mother worries all the time. She sometimes calls me twice a day to check in on me. She knows I am having a rough time." Her father has a cardiac history and experienced a myocardial infarct about 2 years ago. "He was in the cardiac intensive care unit and had a triple bypass performed. He is recovered and is back at work now." Her father, according to Kesha, is a bit of a workaholic who has had to change his lifestyle secondary to the cardiac episode. "He has had to learn how to relax and not work 80 plus hours per week. My mother ran the show when I was growing up. He was never home." She describes that her siblings, Tom and Bob, have no known history of mood or anxiety disorders. Tom is a police officer in the town that we grew up in, and Bob works for the electric company in New York City.

I then proceeded to ask Kesha about the stressors in her life, good and bad, and her reaction to them if she could remember. Kesha denies any significant response to any events in her early childhood. She went to the neighborhood school, had a best friend Whitney, and remembers when her brothers were born, more specifically Bob. "He is 7 years younger than me." She remembers her maternal grandmother coming to stay with them. "That was great. I really love my grandmother, and she is so funny. I remember my parents going off to the hospital, and that night we went with my Dad to visit my mom and Bob. I just wanted to hold him."

In high school, Kesha remembers that she would get a little anxious around test times. "I put up very high expectations of myself. I wanted to get all As, so I would get a little be nervous when I had to take tests. I still do get a bit anxious when something significant is going to happen." She described good interpersonal relationships in high school. "Whitney and I are still friends to this day, even though we live 500 miles apart." She had boyfriends—"nothing serious"—played on sport teams, and was in the choir. She went to college in the Boston area, "and I really never went home. I love Boston." College was described as a "fun time." She majored in biology. She works as a research assistant in one of the hospitals in the Boston area. Her partner, Sam, is a sound engineer and works with one of the television studios in the area. They have been living together for 5 years and planned the pregnancy. "We are doing it all backward. We are getting married in 6 months." She worked until she went into labor, had a 4-month maternity leave because of the family leave legislation, and had been back at work since she was 5 months postpartum. The baby is in the daycare center in the building that houses the laboratory that she works at. "It is a great arrangement. I get to go down and see her whenever I get a break, and we go to work together and go home together. Sam's hours are a bit chaotic at times. It works out well with her at my work place. He is a great dad and involved in her care when he is at home, very different than my father when I was growing up."

I asked Kesha to describe for me her reproductive, labor and delivery history. Kesha experienced menarche at the age of 14 and denies any major issues or concerns with her cycle. "I am regular, every 30 days like clock work. I don't remember any problems with cramps, headaches, bowel changes." She described that she was on oral contraceptives for 6 years with no problems and that she had discontinued them about 4 months before she conceived. "We were very lucky; it didn't take too long to get pregnant, and I felt like I had given my body some time off after being on those pills for so long." Currently, she is back on birth control pills and has not had any problems with them. "But I don't know what else is happening. I have just become so anxious, so worried. I am afraid of everything."

We moved to the pregnancy experience. Kesha described that the first trimester was fine. "I had morning sickness, and I was tired but also so happy to be pregnant. It went away, and then it was fine." Her second trimester was uneventful, as was her third. As we began to speak about her labor and delivery experience, there was a significant change in Kesha's way of being in the room. She began to shake her right leg. Her head went down. Her voice changed, and there were long moments of silence. I gently asked Kesha what she was feeling and what was going on. She looked up at me, tears welling in her eyes. "Do we have to go there?" she asked. "I had a healthy baby; she is fine. Do we need to talk about that day?" I shifted in my chair, gently handed Kesha the box of tissues, and said, "Kesha, I get the feeling that that something happened during that labor and delivery that is causing strong feelings inside of you. Can you share it with me?" My sense at this time, from her positional and affective changes, was that Kesha had experienced some level of trauma in that experience, and she had suppressed her feelings and moved into a coping strategy of "get on with your life." Sadly, I have heard from too many health care providers that same thought: "She had a baby, and the baby is fine. Wasn't that the outcome that everyone wanted? What is she still crying about?" Having a baby is for many women almost like a near-death experience in that she moves from one part of her self to another. Too often there is the push to move on and not process the events that occur in one's life and to just "be happy." My sense was that this therapy with Kesha was going to take a little time in that she had denied her feelings secondary to whatever had happened at that birth, and those feelings were coming through, whether she liked it or not. The brain is an amazing organ. It encodes and takes in every experience in our lives whether we do or not, and those experiences come back as feelings, thoughts, smells, and so forth, when they need to be felt and experienced. Perhaps, at 1 year postpartum, Kesha was able to begin to touch that event. Maybe it was the thoughts of getting married, another major life event, that were triggering these feelings. I knew that to help Kesha she would have to develop a strong rapport with me. Then she could feel safe enough in my office and with me to disclose this very personal experience.

Kesha looked up at me and told me that the birth of her daughter was the "worst experience in my whole life. I have not really talked about it with anyone. I just moved on and tried to live life. She was alive, and I was alive. What was there to worry about?" My internal response was one of intense sadness and a bit aggravated, as that is the way the culture supported traumatic events—move on, get over it. You are still alive. We do not as a culture encourage the verbalization of the experience, the necessity of processing the emotions and the event to be able to honor the emotions and integrate the experience. As Cheryl Beck so eloquently wrote in her article on birth trauma, "Beauty is not the only quality or phenomenon that lies in the eye of the beholder; birth trauma also does. What a mother perceives as birth trauma may be seen quite differently through the eyes of obstetric care providers, who may view it as a routine delivery and just another day at the hospital" (Beck, 2004a, p. 28). I knew that I had to find out what her experience was from her eyes, "the eyes of the beholder."

Kesha looked up hesitantly at me, and I gently smiled and softly stated, "If you can, Kesha, tell me your story. Begin where you feel comfortable, and I will listen." Kesha picked up a few tissues from the box, repositioned herself on the couch, and took a deep breath. She began to tell me her story.

Kesha had experienced the passing of her mucus plug on a Friday evening, and she remembered that the childbirth educator said that labor could start after that but to try and just go on with your day. Kesha and Sam were at home that evening; thus, they just hung around and went to bed early. "We figured we would need the rest and sleep 'cause we would be meeting our baby soon." She slept until about 4:00 a.m. "I awoke with a strong cramp. It jolted me out of my sleep. I got up, went to the bathroom, and noticed that when I wiped there was a moderate amount of bloody show. So I went back to bed and lay there." Within an hour she began to feel contractions, and they were "twinging" about every 20 minutes, "but I wasn't worried at all because that is what they told us would happen." She did not wake Sam but rather just relaxed and did cleansing breaths. "I was getting a bit excited and at the same time nervous. I figured today would be the day that we met our baby. We did not know the sex, so we were really looking forward to the whole process." By 9:00 a.m., "my contractions were coming about every 10 minutes, and they were getting very strong. I was still having that discharge, but I didn't think that my membranes had ruptured." They decided to contact the doctor and let him know what was going on. When the doctor called them back, she was having strong contractions. "They were really focused in my back. I kept trying to lean against the door knobs for counter pressure." The doctor told them to come to the hospital, and he would meet them in labor and delivery. "We were so excited. We were running around the apartment trying to find the things we needed, even though I was very organized and my bag had been packed for 2 weeks!"

Kesha was admitted to the labor and delivery suites and got into bed, and they examined her. "I was about 4 centimeters, and I was having severe backaches. They kept telling me that the contractions would come around the front, but they were not moving. I wanted to have an unmedicated birth, but at that time, I thought I may have to get some medication if I was only 4 cm and I was in that much pain. I tried walking and getting on my hands and knees, which helped a lot." After 3 more hours of intense pain, she describes that she had not progressed very far; thus, they decided to rupture her membranes to see whether that would help the progress. It was after this procedure that someone noted that her baby was in a posterior position, which meant that her head was pushing against her coccyx and that "she would have to turn in utero to let her head come out first, not her face."

"Jeanne, the pain was becoming intense, and they would come and go; no one stayed with us in the room." At one point, I said to Sam, "I don't think I can do this. I need some medication." She describes that Sam was looking a bit anxious himself, and when the doctor came in, she told him that she had changed her mind. She now thought that she would like the epidural. He said he would get the anesthesiologist; he left, and Sam and Kesha were all alone. They were watching the fetal monitor, and they were really working hard with their breathing and focus. All of a sudden, the monitor alarms started to beep. "We didn't know what was happening. We looked at each other, and no one was coming in. It looked like the heart rate had gone down, but we weren't sure. The alarm kept ringing, and still no one came in. Finally, Sam went out of the room and got someone. When the nurse came in she played with the fetoscope, trying to move it around to find the baby's heartbeat. She had a very serious look on her face, but she wasn't saying anything. Then she left. The next thing we knew there were about 10 people in the room, and they told me that the baby was in distress and that they had to take me to the operating room for an emergency caesarean. I remember feeling as cold as ice. I looked at Sam, and then they wheeled me away."

In the operating room, there was a mad rush to get her onto the table. "There were people all over the place. I was freezing and just kept wondering what was going on. Would I die? Would my baby die? Where was Sam?" They told her that they were going to give her general anesthesia and put her to sleep. "I panicked. I was afraid I was going to suffocate. They must have given me something in my intravenous because I started to feel really groggy and foggy. Then I felt this mask go over my face and this intense searing pain in my belly. I thought I had been stabbed, and then I guess I went to sleep because I don't remember anything until a few hours later in recovery room. I woke up, and Sam was at my head, patting and rubbing my arm. I looked at him. I was terrified. I asked him whether the baby was dead, and he looked at me surprised and said, "She is fine, how are you?"

Kesha went on to tell me that she believed that her baby was dead even though Sam said she was fine. "I hadn't seen her yet, and the last I remembered was intense pain and terror." It turned out that the baby was in the NICU, as she had aspirated some meconium. It seemed that she was posterior, and when she began to turn in utero, she was compressing the umbilical cord and cutting down the oxygen so that her heart rate would drop and then she would stop turning. She was in the intensive care for observation and to have antibiotics administered as a result of the aspiration. They wanted to watch her respirations, although they told both Sam and Kesha that the baby was fine.

Kesha started to cry as she told the story, and at this point, she was sobbing. "I thought my baby would be dead, or better yet brain damaged. I had done everything I was supposed to do and look what happened. What did I do to cause that?" I sat there feeling that sense that we as women tend to believe that so much is our fault, that we have the power to control so many things; of course, we don't. This was one issue that Kesha and I might have to address—guilt regarding what she had power over and what she did not.

I asked Kesha to continue the story and tell me about that first day after the caesarean birth. "I had so much pain. I just couldn't get comfortable. I was transferred to my room from the recovery room, and the baby was going to be coming up from the NICU. I just wanted to sleep. I think I was so scared to see her." After she got settled in her room, the baby was brought in. Sam was there, too. Kesha described that the baby looked okay. "She had a hat on her head, and she was awake. I really noticed her eyes. They handed her to me, and I looked at her and just started to cry. Gradually, I begin to touch her face, lay her gently on the pillow on my lap, and undress her. I wanted to make sure that she was intact and had all of her toes and fingers. She was perfect. She did have a little intravenous line in her arm that was for the antibiotics. However, she was fine and kept looking at me. It was so good to see that she was okay. Although, to be honest with you, Jeanne, I kept wondering what had happened to her brain, whether she would have any problems—after all, her heart rate had gone down, and she was delivered by an emergency caesarean section." Here was an issue that Kesha had been holding in her heart since her baby's birth that I would bring up later. So much of my job as a nurse psychotherapist is collecting the dynamic information and the potential psychiatric implications to each individual's coping strategies. Kesha went on telling me about that first day. "The baby really looked at me, and I told her how sorry I was that the birth had to happen that way. It made me so sad that it had become such a rush and in my mind a death-like event. No one ever asked me how it had been for me. It is amazing how the attention all goes to moving on and taking care of the baby and, of course, my incision. The incision is my reminder of the event; Jeanne, it sucks!" I asked Kesha whether she had spoken to anyone about her experience on the delivery table when she felt that searing pain before the mask being put on her face by the anesthesiologist. "No, this is really the first time that I have told anyone. I realized very early that I was supposed to move on and get on with taking care of the baby. I had so much pain for the longest time. I think that there were times when they thought I was an addict. I couldn't get comfortable, and the nurse would remind me regularly that I had to wait for 4 hours for my next pain pill. I just wanted to crawl into a cave and hide, but I had to take care of the baby." I realized that so far she had not called her baby by name but referred to her as the baby. I looked at Kesha and asked her what her daughter's name was. She smiled and said, "Lindsey." I began to wonder what the relationship between Kesha and Lindsey was like. She had come to this visit without her daughter, another area for more information at a later date.

Kesha said that the days in the hospital were hard because she had a lot of pain and the breastfeeding was a bit difficult. "I couldn't get in a comfortable position with the incision. We did eventually get the hang of that. I really ended up liking the breastfeeding, as I felt that that was one good thing that I could do for her since I couldn't even birth her vaginally." Here is another guilt implication: she feels she did not birth well. "I breastfed Lindsey until she was 6 months old. When I went back to work, it was too hard to pump regularly, so we weaned. That was okay with me. She had been having a bottle given to her by Sam since she was about 4 weeks old, so we didn't have any problems with the weaning. I feel like that was a good thing that we had."

I asked Kesha if or when she began to feel that she had recovered from the birth experience. She looked at me and said, "You know, I thought I had recovered, but lately I am a mess. I don't know what is causing these nightmares, the anxiety, the stomach aches, and headaches. I wake up sweating in the middle of the night. I dream that there is a table saw coming at me and I have to wake up so that it won't hurt me." I wondered about this metaphor—a table saw and the searing pain that she experienced when the caesarean was begun. I asked her whether she thought there might be some connection. She looked up and her eyes were stunning, "I never thought about that. I bet they are related. Do you think?" I said that I did indeed think that everything was related.

Kesha went on to describe an uneventful postpartum. "After Lindsey was about 6 months and she was developmentally on target, I began to believe that she was fine and that maybe I could believe my doctor that she had not had any problem with loss of oxygen when she was born. I find that as she gets older I am less worried about that, as she is doing everything she is supposed to do. The daycare people tell me that she is very smart and talks a lot for a baby her age. I figure that they are experts. Why would they lie to me? In many ways, I am feeling better about her, but to be honest with you, I don't know whether she will ever have a sibling. I am terrified to get pregnant again."

I looked at Kesha and shared with her that I thought she was experiencing anxiety symptoms in response to a PTSD secondary to the birth experience and that she had repressed her feelings about the experience until now, as she was coming on the 1-year anniversary. (See Figure 8.1.) The feelings were surging from within. I shared with her that I believe that the feelings have a way of telling us that they need to be honored, felt, named, and integrated. Her experience of the birth was traumatic. She was afraid that she would die and that her baby would die, and when she was alive, the focus went to the area of potential brain damage for Lindsey. I felt that if she was comfortable with me that our therapy would focus on feeling those feelings, in essence working them through. When they were integrated into her ability to self-strategize, she could decide what to do next with regard to having another baby. I felt that she needed to have a good night's sleep and that we could begin with the use of antianxiety medications; however, if she did not feel like she was feeling any better, we could try an antidepressant agent, which has been approved for anxiety and PTSD treatment. Thus, we developed the following NURSE Program (Sichel & Driscoll, 1999).

- **N:** Nutrition and Needs: Kesha described a nutritionally balanced diet, with adequate fluids and protein. She took a multivitamin and calcium supplement daily. I suggested that she begin to take omega-3 fatty acids, vitamin E, and vitamin C, as that had been shown to be helpful in mood and anxiety treatment as a nutritional supplement (Altshuler et al., 2002). We discussed weekly supportive psychotherapy sessions for at least eight sessions, and then we could reevaluate

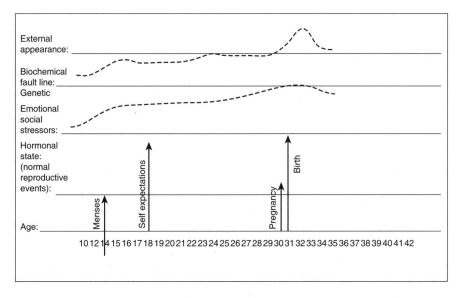

Figure 8.1 The Earthquake Assessment: Kesha
Sichel, D. & Driscoll, J. W. *Women's Moods: What every woman must know about hormones, the brain, and emotional health.* 1999. By permission of HarperCollins Publishers, Inc., p. 100.

the relationship. I discussed the use of low-dose antianxiety medication, which would provide immediate relief of her anxiety symptoms and may help with her sleep. I discussed with her the use of these agents in the beginning, and if we learned that the symptoms were not going away, we might add a specific serotonergic reuptake inhibitor, as they are useful in the treatment of anxiety and depression.

- **U:** Understanding: I gave Kesha some reprints of the article by Cheryl pertaining to birth trauma as a way to validate her experience and for her to feel that she was not alone in her feelings and her thoughts. I like to use articles or handouts if I can because it validates feelings, and women can read the materials more than once. I also encouraged Kesha to begin a journal to write the dreams that she was having as well as anything that came up in response to our therapy together.

- **R:** Rest and relaxation: Kesha described that she was having problems with sleep: inability to get to sleep, nightmares, and not feeling rested after wakening. I prescribed a low dose of clonazepam (Klonopin), 0.5 mg at bedtime, to see whether that would help calm the biochemistry and allow her to have a more restful sleep. I also suggested that she take some Klonopin during the day, starting at 0.5 mg tablet and increasing to one tablet every 6 to 8 hours as needed. My primary goal was to quiet down some of the biology so that she would feel more in control. If she was not sleeping any better after a few nights, I would consider adding an antidepressant to cover her better.

- **S:** Spirituality: Kesha felt that she was comfortable with her own sense of spirituality and prayer was helpful to her.

- **E:** Exercise: Kesha was used to doing an aerobics class three times per week, so I encouraged her to continue that program.

We discussed the care plan, went over the recommendations, and set up a meeting for the next week. She was encouraged to call me with any concerns and to remember that I did not consider any questions or concerns silly or stupid. She seemed more relaxed, and said that she was glad that she had come to see me, was comfortable with me, and looked forward to seeing me the next week.

Kesha came in the next week. She had had some good results with the use of Klonopin but did not feel significantly better. She still felt a bit down and unhappy. The sleep was better, but she was still having some nightmares. We decided to add an SSRI agent to the plan so that she could eventually have better coverage. My thought was that there was a level of depression that was slowly being uncovered as she came to trust me.

The therapy focused on helping her to mourn the birth experience, to validate her perceptive reality, and to make peace with what had been. Over our time together, Kesha made significant strides in her healing. She continued on an antidepressant agent with the occasional use of the antianxiety agent. She was planning her wedding and was even able to consider having another baby. However, she was very verbal in the idea that she would want to speak with her obstetrician regarding the past delivery experience and was considering an elective cesarean so that she did not have to worry about another traumatic labor and delivery experience. That issue was to be ongoing in our work together.

The recovery from a posttraumatic experience secondary to a birth trauma requires time and what I call being a nurse-midwife to the process. A trusted listener, able to witness and support the personal and perceptive reality of the woman and her experience, is a necessary aspect of the healing journey. She needs to experience the grieving process as she mourns the loss of what happened to her. The outcome may have been positive—mother and baby were alive—but the process was horrific.

References

Allen, S. (1998). A qualitative analysis of the process, mediating variables and impact of traumatic childbirth. *Journal of Reproductive and Infant Psychology*, 16, 107–131.

Altshuler, L. L., Cohen, L. S., Moline, M. L., Kahn, D. A., Carpenter, D., Docherty, J. P., et al. (2002). Expert consensus guidelines for the treatment of depression in women: A new treatment tool. *MentalFitness*, 1(1), 69–83.

American Psychiatric Association. (1980). *Diagnostic and statistical manual of mental disorders*. Washington, DC: Author.

American Psychiatric Association. (2000). *Diagnostic and statistical manual of mental disorders* (4th ed., text revision). Washington, DC: author.

American Psychological Association. (1994). *Diagnostic and statistical manual of mental disorders* (4th ed.). Washington, DC: Author.

Ayers, S., & Pickering, A. (2001). Do women get posttraumatic stress disorder as a result of childbirth? A prospective study of incidence. *Birth*, 28, 111–118.

Beck, C. T. (2004a). Birth trauma: In the eye of the beholder. *Nursing Research*, 53(1), 28–35.

Beck, C. T. (2004b). Posttraumatic stress disorder due to childbirth: The aftermath. *Nursing research*, 53, 216–224.

Callahan, J. L., & Hynan, M. T. (2002). Identifying mothers at risk for postnatal emotional distress: Further evidence for the validity of the Perinatal Posttraumatic Stress Disorder Questionnaire. *Journal of Perinatology*, 22, 448–454.

Chrousos, G. P., Torpy, D. J., & Gold, P. W. (1998). Interactions between the hypothalamic–pituitary–adrenal axis and the female reproductive system: Clinical implications. *Annals of Internal Medicine*, 129(3), 229–234.

Church, S., & Scanlan, M. (2002). Post-traumatic stress disorder after childbirth. *The Practicing Midwife*, 5, 10–13.

Cohen, M. M., Ansara, D., Schei, B., Stuckless, N., & Stewart, D.(2004). Posttraumatic stress disorder after pregnancy labor and delivery. *Journal of Women's Health*, 13, 315–324.

Creedy, D. K., Shochet, I. M., & Horsfall, J. (2000). Childbirth and the development of acute trauma symptoms: Incidence and contributing factors. *Birth*, 27, 104–111.

Crompton, J. (1996). Post-traumatic stress disorder and childbirth: 2. *British Journal of Midwifery*, 4, 354–356.

Czarnocka, J., & Slade, P.(2000), Prevalence and predictors of posttraumatic stress symptoms following childbirth. *British Journal of Clinical Psychology*, 39, 35–51.

Davidson, J., & Connor, K. M. (1999). Management of posttraumatic stress disorder: Diagnostic and therapeutic issues. *Journal of Clinical Psychiatry*, 60(Suppl. 18), 33–38.

Davidson, J. R. T., Book, S. W., Colket, J. T., & Tupler, L. A. (1997) Assessment of a new self-rating scale for posttraumatic stress disorder. *Psychological Medicine*, 27, 153.

DeMier, R. L., Hynan, M. T., Harris, H. B., & Manniello, R. L. (1996). Perinatal stressors as predictors of symptoms of posttraumatic stress in mothers of infants at high risk. *Journal of Perinatology*, 16, 276–280.

Foa, E. B., Riggs, D. S., Dancu, C., & Rothbaum, B. O. (1993). Reliability and validity of a brief instrument for assessing posttraumatic stress disorder. *Journal of Trauma Stress*, 6, 459–473.

Hendrick, V., & Gitlin, M. J. (2004). *Psychotropic drugs and women: Fast facts*. New York: W. W. Norton & Company.

Holditch-Davis, D., Bartlett, T. R., Blickman, A. L., & Miles, M. S. (2003). Posttraumatic stress symptoms in mothers of premature infants. *Journal of Obstetric, Gynecologic, and Neonatal Nursing*, 32, 161–171.

Horowitz, M. J., Wilner, N., & Alvarez, W. (1979). Revised Impact of Event Scale: A measure of subjective stress. *Psychosomatic Medicine*, 41, 209–218.

Kennedy, H.P., & MacDonald, E.L. (2002). "Altered consciousness" during childbirth: Potential clues to post-traumatic stress disorder? *Journal of Midwifery and Women's Health*, 47, 380–381.

Lyons, S. (1998). A prospective study of posttraumatic stress symptoms 1 month following childbirth in a group of 42 first-time mothers. *Journal of Reproductive and Infant Psychology*, 16, 91–105.

Marshall, R. D., & Pierce, D. (2000). Implications of recent findings in posttraumatic stress disorder and the role of pharmacotherapy. *Harvard Review of Psychiatry*, 7(5), 247–256.

Menage, J. (1993). Post-traumatic stress disorder in women who have undergone obstetric or gynecological procedures. *Journal of Reproduction and Infant Psychology*, 11, 221–228.

Pigott, T. A. (2002). Anxiety disorders. In S. G. Kornstein & A. H. Clayton (Eds.), *Women's Mental Health: A comprehensive textbook* (pp. 195–221). New York: The Guilford Press.

Rothbaum, B. O., Ninan, P. T., & Thomas, L. (1996). Sertraline in the treatment of rape victims with posttraumatic stress disorder. *Journal of Trauma and Stress*, 9(4), 865–871.

Ryding, E.L., Wijma, K., & Wijma, B. (1998). Psychological impact of emergency cesarean section in comparison with elective cesarean section, instrumental, and normal vaginal delivery. *Journal of Psychosomatic Obstetrics and Gynecology*, 19, 135–144.

Sichel, D. A., & Driscoll, J. W. (1999). *Women's moods: What every woman must know about the hormones, the brain, and emotional health*. New York: William Morrow Publishers.

Soet, J. E., Brack, G. A., & Dilorio, C. (2003). Prevalence and predictors of women's experience of psychological trauma during childbirth. *Birth*, 30, 36–46.

Watson, C. C., Juba, M. P., Manifold, V., Kucala, T., & Anderson, E. D. (1991). The PTSD Interview: Rationale, description, reliability, and concurrent validity of a DSM-III-based technique. *Journal of Clinical Psychology*, 47, 179–189.

Wijma, K., Soderquist, M. A., & Wijma, B. (1997). Posttraumatic stress disorder after childbirth: A cross sectional study. *Journal of Anxiety Disorders*, 11, 587–597.

CHAPTER 9

SCREENING INSTRUMENTS

In this chapter, instruments are discussed that can be used to screen for postpartum depression, risk factors for postpartum depression, maternity blues, posttraumatic stress disorder (PTSD) caused by childbirth, bipolar II disorder, and obsessive compulsive disorder.

Postpartum Depression

One of the most difficult challenges in dealing with postpartum depression has been early recognition (Harberger, Berchtold, & Honikman, 1992). A striking feature of this mood disorder is how covertly it is experienced. Because this postpartum mood disorder often goes unrecognized by clinicians, mothers in the community suffer in silence, fear, and confusion because they have not been diagnosed. Undiagnosed postpartum depression can result in tragedy—not always in the form of maternal suicide or infanticide that one reads in the headlines. It can plunge mothers into the depths of despair and turn their first months of motherhood into blackness.

Approximately 400,000 mothers in America experience this postpartum mood disorder each year, most often 6 to 8 weeks after delivery (Kleiman & Raskin, 1994). Clinicians only identify a small percentage of these mothers, however, as depressed. Hearn et al. (1998) reported that despite an average of 14 healthcare contacts with each of the 176 mothers in the postpartum period, almost half of the women who were depressed had not been identified as such by the clinicians.

Mothers with postpartum depression may not seek treatment because of a lack of knowledge about this mood disorder or because of the tremendous stigma. They may fear that if they show their feelings, child welfare authorities may take their infants.

Holopainen (2001) conducted a qualitative study of postpartum depressed women in Australia and their experiences in seeking help for their depression. Most of the mothers revealed that they did not know how or when to seek help. These mothers realized that something was wrong with them, but they did not actively seek help because they did not know that they were experiencing postpartum depression. When these women did receive professional help, it was mainly incidental, and they were identified by maternal health nurses during a baby checkup.

In Iceland, mothers with elevated depressive symptomatology shared the reasons why, even though they were severely distressed, they did not seek health care (Thome, 2003). These reasons fell into five categories: (1) inappropriate institution to treat mental, emotional, and spiritual problems, (2) a lack of appropriate assessment of how people feel, (3) a lack of expert professional care in treatment of mental health problems, (4) a lack of professional distance between patient and health professional, and (5) misinterpretation of depressive symptoms.

MacLennan, Wilson, and Taylor (1996) interviewed 1,102 mothers who had recently given birth and indicated that only 49% of those women who felt seriously depressed had sought help for their depression. Compounding this tragic problem is the fact that health care providers tend to minimize the seriousness of postpartum depression and equate it simply with maternity blues. Also, clinicians do not want to dwell on the dark side of motherhood (Huysman, 1998).

England, Ballard, and George (1994) found that the longer the delay from onset of postpartum depression to the beginning of adequate antidepressant/psychologic interventions, the longer the duration of this mood disorder, which usually lasts more than 6 months. This finding highlights the need for early diagnosis and treatment of postpartum depression.

In Canada at 1, 4, and 8 weeks postpartum, mothers with depressive symptoms had a significantly higher number of contacts with health care providers than nondepressed mothers (Dennis, 2004). Mothers with depressive symptoms at 4 weeks after giving birth reported that the care they received from their family physicians was unhelpful. Dennis suggested that clinicians should screen for postpartum depression when they have a patient who is frequently using health services.

Postpartum depression is treatable, but before this can happen, women suffering from it must be identified. Routine screening of new mothers for this crippling mood disorder is imperative. Women need to be screened periodically throughout the first 12 months after delivery. Screening once is not enough if a mother screens negative, indicating that she is not currently experiencing high levels of postpartum depressive symptoms. Just because a mother screens negative at one point in time, for example, 6-weeks postpartum, it does not mean that she could not develop postpartum depression sometime later during the first year after delivery.

Screening is not just the responsibility of clinicians in the field of obstetrics. In fact, mothers lose contact with their nurse-midwives and obstetricians usually after the 6-week postpartum checkup unless they are having some physical problems. A mother's next scheduled visit usually is at 1 year after delivery for a routine pap smear. For the majority of mothers, their most consistent ongoing contact with a health care provider during the first year after delivery will be with clinicians in the field of pediatrics and family practice, such as pediatric nurse practitioners and pediatricians. Primary care clinicians also may have contact with new mothers, but not as consistently as pediatricians. Screening mothers for postpartum depression at well-baby checkups is an ideal opportunity.

Pediatricians are on the front lines to screen mothers for postpartum depression. Wiley, Burke, Gill, and Law (2004) assessed 389 pediatricians' knowledge and views regarding postpartum depression. Only 31% of the pediatricians felt confident that they would be able to recognize whether a mother was suffering from postpartum depression. Only 7% of the pediatricians were familiar with screening scales for this postpartum mood disorder. Approximately half (49%) of the pediatricians reported they had little or no education about this mood disorder. Female pediatricians and younger pediatricians were more likely to screen for postpartum depression.

In recent focus groups, mothers revealed that they trusted their pediatricians with the health of their children, but many mothers hesitated to share their depressive symptoms with their child's pediatrician (Heneghan, Mercer, & DeLeone, 2004). Mothers feared that they would be judged and that a possible referral to child protection service would be made if they talked with their pediatrician about their depressive symptoms. Trust and open communication with their pediatricians were considered vital to the mothers' willingness to discuss their depressive symptoms. All women's health care providers must bear the responsibility of their role in screening mothers for postpartum depression. An interdisciplinary approach is ideal, including nursing, medicine, social work, mental health, pediatrics, family, and community support systems.

In screening, health care professionals must be aware that women who are experiencing postpartum depression may find it difficult to confide their feelings to others. One reason for this hesitancy is the popular myth that equates becoming a mother with happiness. New motherhood is idealized in our society. Joy and other positive feelings are emphasized, whereas sadness and other negative emotions are minimized. It is culturally acceptable to be depressed after a death, divorce, or job loss, but not by the arrival of an infant (Gruen, 1990). Because of the social stigma surrounding depression after delivery, mothers may experience shame, fear, or embarrassment in sharing their negative feelings.

Before asking mothers about their experiences with postpartum depression, clinicians need to dispel this cultural myth and give mothers permission to speak about any negative feelings that they might be experiencing. Clinicians can share with new mothers the concept that childbirth and early motherhood also can be viewed from Jeanne's framework of loss and grief (Driscoll, 1990). In postpartum depression, loss is an important theme. The mother may experience a loss of energy, self, relationships, social roles, and lifestyle.

Postpartum Depression Screening Scale

The Postpartum Depression Screening Scale (PDSS) was developed by Beck and Gable (2002). It is a 35-item self-report scale that is designed to assess the presence, severity, and type of postpartum depression symptoms (Table 9.1). The PDSS screens for this devastating mental illness by identifying women who have a high probability of meeting diagnostic criteria for a depressive disorder with postpartum onset, as defined by the *Diagnostic and Statistical Manual of Mental Disorder, Fourth Edition-Text Revision* (DSM-IV-TR; American Psychiatric Association, 2000). The PDSS yields a total score, which indicates the overall severity of postpartum depressive symptoms and helps to determine whether the woman needs to be referred for additional diagnostic evaluation. The PDSS consists of seven symptom content subscales and also provides an inconsistent responding index as an indicator of response validity. The PDSS items are written at a third-grade reading level. The items consist of statements about how a mother may be feeling after the birth of her baby. A 5-point Likert response format (1 = strongly disagree, 5 = strongly agree) is used. Because all items are negatively worded, agreement with an item constitutes endorsement of the depressive symptom. Higher scores on the PDSS indicate higher levels of postpartum depressive symptoms, whereas lower scores indicate lower levels of these symptoms and suggest a relatively normal postpartum adjustment.

Table 9.1   POSTPARTUM DEPRESSION SCREENING SCALE:
SELECTED ITEMS BY DIMENSION

During the past 2 weeks I. . .

Sleeping/Eating Disturbances
#1: I had trouble sleeping even when my baby was asleep.
#8: I lost my appetite.

Loss of Self
#19: I did not know who I was anymore.
#5: I was afraid that I would never by my normal self again.

Anxiety/Insecurity
#23: I felt all alone.
#9: I felt really overwhelmed.

Guilt/Shame
#20: I felt guilty because I could not feel as much love for my baby as I should.
#27: I felt like I had to hide what I was thinking or feeling toward the baby.

Emotional Lability
#3: I felt like my emotions were on a roller coaster.
#31: I felt full of anger ready to explode.

Mental Confusion
#11: I could not concentrate on anything.
#4: I felt like I was losing my mind.

Suicidal Thoughts
#14: I started thinking I would be better off dead.
#28: I felt that my baby would be better off without me.

Because this postpartum mood disorder is not a homogenous one, different women may experience varying constellations of symptoms, which in turn need different treatment approaches. The PDSS was designed to measure seven symptom content areas that individual women may experience. The PDSS symptom content scales were derived from Cheryl's qualitative research studies on the subjective experience of postpartum depression (Beck, 1992, 1993, 1996). The seven content scales are as follows: sleeping/eating disturbances, anxiety/insecurity, emotional lability, mental confusion, loss of self, guilt/shame, and suicidal thoughts. The PDSS yields a separate score for each of the seven scales, and its manual provides guidelines for interpreting elevations on these scales (Beck & Gable, 2002).

Screening for postpartum depression requires sensitivity on the part of clinicians. Women who experience this mood disorder may find it difficult to confide their feelings because of social stigmas surrounding depression after the birth of a baby. To begin, a clinician may also want to discuss the mother's expectations and reactions to her role of new motherhood. Often mothers believe the myth that new motherhood should lead to all positive emotions, and they may be hesitant to disclose feelings that do not fit with these ideals. By gently "normalizing" the wide range of feelings, both positive and negative, that often accompany new motherhood, a health care provider can help the mother to complete the screening scale in an open and honest manner.

PDSS Total Scores

The PDSS total score is based on responses to all 35 items and has a possible range of 35 to 175 (see Table 9.1). It provides an index of the severity of a mother's postpartum depressive symptoms. The PDSS total score is interpreted by means of three ranges: normal adjustment, significant symptoms of postpartum depression, and a positive screen for major postpartum depression (Beck & Gable, 2002).

Scores in the range of normal adjustment indicate a lack of significant symptoms of postpartum depression. Mothers who score in this range usually do not need to be referred to psychiatric evaluation, unless of course there is evidence of significant depression or other psychopathology from another source of information. Clinicians should provide women who attain scores in this normal adjustment range with basic information regarding postpartum depression so that they can be alert to these symptoms in case later in their postpartum period they start to experience any of them. Beck and Gable (2002) recommended readministering the

PDSS every 3 months during the first 12 months after delivery to provide continued screening for postpartum depression.

Women who score in the range of significant symptoms of postpartum depression tend to be experiencing minor depression. Some of the mothers scoring in this range may need to be referred for formal psychiatric evaluation. In deciding whether to refer a mother in this range for further evaluation, the health care provider must consider additional sources of information, such as the mother's medical and psychiatric history, the results of other psychologic tests, the evaluations of other clinicians, and interviews with significant others. If there is evidence that the mother poses a danger to herself or to others, she must be referred immediately for psychiatric evaluation.

If the clinician decides not to refer a mother in this range for psychiatric evaluation, information should be given to the mother about what to do if her symptoms should worsen (e.g., how to access specialists in the treatment of postpartum depression). It is also helpful to provide the mother with a list of local new mother and postpartum depression support groups. Finally, it is advisable to readminister the PDSS to the mother at her subsequent contacts with the health care system during the first 12 months after delivery.

Scores in the range of a positive screen for major postpartum depression indicate a high probability that the mother is suffering from this disorder. Mothers who score in this range are in definite need of psychiatric evaluation and should be referred as soon as possible to the mental health team for further assessment and treatment. If there is indication of danger to self (e.g., elevation on the PDSS Suicidal Thoughts scale) or to others, the mother should be referred immediately to emergency department psychiatric services.

Symptom Content Scores

Whenever the PDSS total score is elevated above the range of normal adjustment, it is helpful to examine the scores for the seven symptom content scales in order to identify the pattern of symptoms for a specific mother. Each symptom content scale is based on five items. The content scales are interpreted by means of ranges of elevation (Beck & Gable, 2002). When a mother scores in the elevated range for a specific content scale, it indicates that she is experiencing substantially more problems in that symptom area than the average mother. The specific ranges of elevation for the seven symptom content scales can be found in the PDSS Manual (Beck & Gable, 2002).

Psychometrics of the PDSS

A sample of 525 mothers (a mean of 6 weeks postpartum) was used to assess the reliability and validity of the PDSS (Beck & Gable, 2000). Cronbach alpha reliabilities for the seven dimensions included the following:

1. Sleeping/eating disturbances (0.83)
2. Anxiety/insecurity (0.83)
3. Emotional lability (0.89)
4. Guilt/shame (0.89)
5. Cognitive impairment (0.91)
6. Suicidal thoughts (0.93)
7. Loss of self (0.94)

Construct validity was examined using confirmatory factor analysis. The standardized weights for the five items per each of the seven dimensions were sufficiently high, indicating that the items fit the hypothesized seven-factor model. Also judged supportive of model fit was the Tucker-Lewis Index of 0.87 and root mean square residual of 0.05.

Further validation of the PDSS was undertaken with a sample of 150 women (mean of 6 weeks postpartum) (Beck & Gable, 2001). Each mother completed the PDSS and was immediately interviewed by a nurse psychotherapist, Jeanne, using the Structured Clinical Interview for DSM-IV Axis 1 Disorders (First, Spitzer, Gibbon, & Williams, 1997) to confirm a suspected DSM-IV diagnosis for major or minor postpartum depressive disorder with postpartum onset. Using receiver operating characteristic curves, a PDSS cut-off score of 80 (sensitivity = 94% and specificity = 98%) is recommended for major PPD, whereas a cut-off score of 60 (sensitivity = 91% and specificity = 72%) is recommended for minor or major depression.

Edinburgh Postnatal Depression Scale

The Edinburgh Postnatal Depression Scale (EPDS) (Cox, Holden, & Sagovsky, 1987) consists of 10 short items of common depressive symptoms. These symptoms include inability to laugh, inability to look forward to things with enjoyment, blaming oneself unnecessarily, feeling anxious or worried, feeling scared or panicky, feeling that "things have been getting on top of me," difficulty sleeping because of unhappiness, feeling sad or miserable, crying, and thoughts of harming oneself. Each item is rated on a scale of 0 to 3. Possible scores can range from 0 to 30. The woman chooses the response that best describes the way that she has been feeling for the past week. With a cutoff of 12/13 for the EPDS, Cox et al. (1987) reported a sensitivity of 86% and a specificity of 78%. The alpha reliability was 0.87. The psychometrics of the EPDS have been assessed in numerous studies. When detecting major depression, its sensitivity has ranged from 67% (Zelkowitz & Millet, 1995) to 100% (Thompson, Harris, Lazarus, & Richards, 1998), and its reported specificity has ranged from 68% (Lawrie, Hofmeyr, de Jager, & Berk, 1998) to 94% (Zelkowitz & Millet, 1995). When detecting minor depression, the reported range of sensitivity was 52% to 73% (Murray & Carothers, 1990). For detection of minor and major depression combined, the EPDS sensitivity ranged from 68% (Murray & Carothers, 1990) to 80% (Lawrie et al., 1998), and its reported specificity was 77% (Lawrie et al., 1998).

Screening Women at Risk for Postpartum Depression

Postpartum Depression Predictors Inventory (PDPI) Revised

"The PDPI-Revised consists of 13 risk factors found to be related to postpartum depression in Beck's (2001) updated meta-analysis (see Table 9.2). All 13 relationships were found to be statistically significant. Guide questions for each predictor that clinicians can use during the interview process are also listed in Table 9.2. These guide questions are intended to assist health care providers in determining whether a risk factor is present in the woman being interviewed. The first 10 risk factors can be assessed during both the prenatal and postpartum periods. After a woman has delivered, the last three predictors—childcare stress, infant temperament, and maternity blues—can be assessed. Two demographic characteristics are now included in the PDPI-Revised: marital status and socioeconomic status. At risk are mothers who are single and have low socioeconomic status.

The PDPI-Revised is not a self-report questionnaire but instead is designed to be administered via an interview conducted by a clinician. The interview format provides a woman with an opportunity to discuss her experiences regarding these risk factors for which interventions can be planned to address each woman's problems. The purpose of the PDPI-Revised results is

Table 9.2   POSTPARTUM DEPRESSION PREDICTORS INVENTORY (PDPI)—
REVISED AND GUIDE QUESTIONS FOR ITS USE

DURING PREGNANCY	CHECK ONE	

Marital Status

Single	❏
Married/cohabitating	❏
Separated	❏
Divorced	❏
Widowed	❏
Partnered	❏

Socioeconomic Status

Low	❏
Middle	❏
High	❏

Self-esteem	Yes	No
Do you feel good about yourself as a person?	❏	❏
Do you feel worthwhile?	❏	❏
Do you feel you have a number of good qualities as a person?	❏	❏

Prenatal Depression

1. Have you ever felt depressed during your pregnancy?	❏	❏

   If yes, when and how long have you been feeling this way?

   If yes, how mild or severe would you consider your depression?

Prenatal Anxiety

1. Have you ever felt anxious during your pregnancy?	❏	❏

   If yes, how long have you been feeling this way?

Unplanned/Unwanted Pregnancy

Was the pregnancy planned?	❏	❏
Is the pregnancy unwanted?	❏	❏

History of Previous Depression

1. Before this pregnancy, have you ever been depressed?	❏	❏

   If yes, when did you experience this depression?

   If yes, have you been under a physician's care for this past depression?

   If yes, did the physician prescribe any medication for your depression?

Social Support

1. Do you feel you receive adequate support from your partner?	❏	❏
2. Do you feel you receive adequate instrumental support from your partner (e.g., help with household chores or babysitting)?	❏	❏

(continues)

Table 9.2 POSTPARTUM DEPRESSION PREDICTORS INVENTORY (PDPI)—
REVISED AND GUIDE QUESTIONS FOR ITS USE

---

3. Do you feel you can rely on your partner when you need help? ❏ ❏
4. Do you feel you can confide in you partner? ❏ ❏
   (repeat the same questions for family and again for friends)

Marital Satisfaction

1. Are you satisfied with your marriage (or living arrangement)? ❏ ❏
2. Are you currently experiencing any marital problems? ❏ ❏
3. Are things going well between you and your partner? ❏ ❏

Life Stress

1. Are you currently experiencing any stressful events
   in your life such as:

   Financial problems ❏ ❏
   Marital problems ❏ ❏
   Death in the family ❏ ❏
   Serious illness in the family ❏ ❏
   Moving ❏ ❏
   Unemployment ❏ ❏
   Job change ❏ ❏

After delivery, add the following items:

Child Care Stress

1. Is your infant experiencing any health problems? ❏ ❏
2. Are you having problems with your baby feeding? ❏ ❏
3. Are you having problems with your baby sleeping? ❏ ❏

Infant Temperament

1. Would you consider your baby irritable or fussy? ❏ ❏
2. Does your baby cry a lot? ❏ ❏
3. Is your baby difficult to console or soothe? ❏ ❏

Maternity Blues

1. Did you experience a brief period of tearfulness and ❏ ❏
   mood swings during the first week after delivery?

Comments:

_____

_____

_____

Reprinted with permission from Beck, Revision of the Postpartum Depression Predictors Inventory.
Journal of Obstetric, Gynecologic, and Neonatal Nursing, 31,339–400, 2002.

not to calculate a cutoff score above which a woman is flagged as at high risk for developing postpartum depression" (Beck, 2002, p. 398, 400).

"Ideally, the PDPI-Revised will be completed once each trimester to update a pregnant woman's risk status. For example, a woman's prenatal anxiety can change from the 2nd to 3rd trimester, and her risk of developing postpartum depression could change accordingly. The PDPI-Revised also should be used periodically after delivery to assess a woman's risk status. She can develop this mood disorder any time during the first 12 months after delivery. Women identified during pregnancy as being at risk for developing postpartum depression should be referred for telephone follow-up after delivery, and if possible, home visits should be made. Nurses should not wait until a woman's 6-week postpartum checkup to assess her status regarding postpartum depression. Some women may need to be referred for psychiatric evaluation for counseling or medication. Suicidal ideation should also be assessed by nurses and immediate emergency measures instituted if present.

Clinicians need to remember, however, that risk indicates only the likelihood that women who are exposed to certain factors (risk factors) will subsequently develop postpartum depression. Risk factors or predictors are characteristics associated with an increased risk of being depressed postpartum. Some risk factors are inherited, whereas others are not. Some risk factors are modifiable, whereas others are not (Harkness, 1995).

Once the modifiable risk factors are identified, clinicians can target interventions to help decrease a woman's risk for developing this mood disorder. Often, a combination of risk factors is identified that places a woman at high risk. Although risk factors are indicators of an increased probability of developing this postpartum mood disorder, they may or may not be directly related to its cause. It is important for clinicians to keep mind, however, that the presence of a risk factor does not necessarily mean that a woman will develop postpartum depression" (Beck, 2002, pp. 400–401).

Screening for Maternity Blues

The Stein Maternity Blues Scale (Stein, 1980) consists of a 13-symptom, self-rating scale. The symptoms listed are depression, crying, anxiety, tension, restlessness, exhaustion, dreaming, appetite, headache, irritability, poor concentration, forgetfulness, and confusion.

Stein's scale provides an overall severity score for each day and also an average score for the entire week. The score for the first eight symptoms is indicated by the number circled. The number of choices for each symptom varies. For example, the choices for the symptom of tension range from 0 to 2: 0 = I feel calm and relaxed, 1 = I feel somewhat tense, and 2 = I feel very tense. The choice for the symptom of crying range from 0 to 4: 0 = I do not feel like crying, 1 = I feel as if I could cry but have not actually cried, 2 = I have shed a few tears today, 3 = I have cried for several minutes today but for less than half an hour, and 4 = I have cried for more than half an hour. Each of the last five symptoms is given a score of 1 if it is present and 0 if it is not. The sum of the scores for all of the symptoms provides the daily score, which can range from 0 to 26. A daily score of 0 to 2 indicates the absence of maternity blues; 3 to 8 is reflective of mild to moderate blues, and 9 or higher indicates severe maternity blues. Acceptable levels of reliability and validity for this scale have been reported (Stein, 1980).

The Blues Questionnaire (Kennerley & Gath, 1989) is a 28-item scale that was devised to detect symptoms of maternity blues (Table 9.3). The items cluster in the following categories: primary blues, retardation, hypersensitivity, decreased self-confidence, depression, reservation, and despondency. Compared with Stein's (1980) scale, the Blues Questionnaire has 18 items/symptoms that do not appear in Stein's questionnaire. Three of the items in Stein's scale (anorexia, dreaming, and headache) are not assessed by the Blues Questionnaire.

The Blues Questionnaire assesses the presence or absence of the 28 blues symptoms. In addition, the 5-point scale ranging from "much less than usual" to "much more than usual" can be used to assess severities of each symptom.

Screening for PTSD After Childbirth

The Perinatal Posttraumatic Stress Disorder Questionnaire (PPQ) is a self-report inventory consisting of 14 yes/no items designed to assess symptoms of PTSD specifically related to childbirth experiences (DeMier, Hyman, Harris, & Manniello, 1996) (Table 9.4). Mothers are asked to answer yes to an item only if the experience listed in that item lasted longer than 1 month during the 6 months after delivery. The first three items focus on symptoms of unwanted intrusions. The next six items identify symptoms of avoidance or numbing of responsiveness. The final five items are specific to symptoms of arousal.

Table 9.3   BLUES QUESTIONNAIRE: KENNERLEY

SUBJECT NAME: _____ NO: _____ DATE: _____ DAYS POSTPARTUM: _____

Below is a list of words that newly delivered mothers have used to describe how they are feeling. Please indicate how you have been feeling today by checking no or yes. Then please mark the box that best describes how much change there is, if any, from your usual self.

	No	Yes	IS THIS	MUCH LESS THAN USUAL	LESS THAN USUAL	NO DIFFERENT	MORE THAN USUAL	MUCH MORE THAN USUAL
1. Tearful	❑	❑		❑	❑	❑	❑	❑
2. Mentally tense	❑	❑		❑	❑	❑	❑	❑
3. Able to concentrate	❑	❑		❑	❑	❑	❑	❑
4. Low spirited	❑	❑		❑	❑	❑	❑	❑
5. Elated	❑	❑		❑	❑	❑	❑	❑
6. Helpless	❑	❑		❑	❑	❑	❑	❑
7. Finding it difficult to show your feelings	❑	❑		❑	❑	❑	❑	❑
8. Alert	❑	❑		❑	❑	❑	❑	❑
9. Forgetful, muddled	❑	❑		❑	❑	❑	❑	❑
10. Anxious	❑	❑		❑	❑	❑	❑	❑
11. Wishing you were alone	❑	❑		❑	❑	❑	❑	❑
12. Mentally relaxed	❑	❑		❑	❑	❑	❑	❑
13. Brooding on things	❑	❑		❑	❑	❑	❑	❑
14. Feeling sorry for yourself	❑	❑		❑	❑	❑	❑	❑
15. Emotionally numb, without feelings	❑	❑		❑	❑	❑	❑	❑
16. Depressed	❑	❑		❑	❑	❑	❑	❑
17. Overemotional	❑	❑		❑	❑	❑	❑	❑
18. Happy	❑	❑		❑	❑	❑	❑	❑
19. Confident	❑	❑		❑	❑	❑	❑	❑
20. Changeable in your spirits	❑	❑		❑	❑	❑	❑	❑
21. Tired	❑	❑		❑	❑	❑	❑	❑

(continues)

Table 9.3   BLUES QUESTIONNAIRE: KENNERLEY (continued)

	No	Yes	IS THIS	Much Less than Usual	Less than Usual	No Different	More than Usual	Much More than Usual
22. Irritable	❑	❑		❑	❑	❑	❑	❑
23. Crying without being able to stop	❑	❑		❑	❑	❑	❑	❑
24. Lively	❑	❑		❑	❑	❑	❑	❑
25. Oversensitive	❑	❑		❑	❑	❑	❑	❑
26. Up and down in your mood	❑	❑		❑	❑	❑	❑	❑
27. Restless	❑	❑		❑	❑	❑	❑	❑
28. Calm, tranquil	❑	❑		❑	❑	❑	❑	❑

Reprinted with permission from Kennerly and Gath, Maternity Blues 1. Detection and measurement by questionnaire. British Journal of Psychiatry, 155, p.362 1989.

Table 9.4   PERINATAL PTSD QUESTIONNAIRE

Please circle "Y" if you had any of the following experiences within 6 months of the birth you just described. Circle "Y" only if the particular experience lasted longer than 1 month during this 6-month period.

Y   N   1. Did you have several bad dreams of giving birth or of your baby's hospital stay?

Y   N   2. Did you have several upsetting memories of giving birth or of your baby's hospital stay?

Y   N   3. Did you have any sudden feelings as though your baby's birth was happening again?

Y   N   4. Did you try to avoid thinking about childbirth or your baby's birth was happening again?

Y   N   5. Did you avoid doing things that might bring up feelings you had about childbirth or your baby's hospital stay (e.g., not watching a TV show about babies)?

Y   N   6. Were you unable to remember parts of your baby's stay?

(continues)

Table 9.4   PERINATAL PTSD QUESTIONNAIRE *(continued)*

Y   N   7. Did you lose interest in doing things you usually do (e.g., did you lose interest in your work or your family)?

Y   N   8. Did you feel alone and removed from other people (e.g., did you feel as if no one understood you)?

Y   N   9. Did it become more difficult for you to feel tenderness or love with others?

Y   N   10. Did you have unusual difficulty falling asleep or staying asleep?

Y   N   11. Were you more irritable or angry with others than usual?

Y   N   12. Did you have greater difficulties concentrating than before you gave birth?

Y   N   13. Did you feel more jumpy (e.g., did you feel more sensitive to noise or more easily startled)?

Y   N   14. Did you feel more guilt about the childbirth than you felt you should have?

Reprinted with permission from DeMier et al., Perinatal stressors as predictors of posttraumatic stress in mothers of infants at high risk. *Journal of Perinatology,* 16, p. 278, 1996).

DeMier et al. (1996) developed the PPQ based on the DSM-111R diagnostic criteria for PTSD and also from an instrument designed to assess PTSD in Israeli soldiers (Solomon, Weisenberg, Scharzwald, & Mikulincer, 1987). The PPQ obtained an alpha coefficient of 0.85 and a test-retest reliability of 0.92 in sample of mothers of high-risk infants and mothers of healthy, full-term infants (DeMier, 1994).

Screening for Bipolar II Disorder

The Mood Disorder Questionnaire (Hirschfeld et al., 2000) is useful as a screening tool to identify bipolar disorder. Although it is not specific for the differentiation between bipolar I and bipolar II, it can help the clinician via the responses of the patient to recognize some aspect of bipolarity. This instrument is based on the DSM-IV criteria for bipolar disorder. It screens for a lifetime history of a hypomanic or manic syndrome with 13 yes/no items. In addition, there is an item that assesses the level of functional impairment caused by these symptoms. Another yes/no item focuses on whether more than one of the symptoms occurred during the same time period. Hirschfeld et al. (2000) reported an internal consistency reliability of 0.90 for the Mood Disorder Questionnaire. A score of seven or more is recommended as the optimal cutoff for screening for bipolar disorder with a sensitivity of 0.73 and a specificity of 0.90.

In 2002, Ronald Pies, clinical professor of psychiatry at Tufts University School of Medicine, developed the Bipolar Spectrum Diagnostic Scale (BSDS) in consultation with Chris Miller, research coordinator of the bipolar disorder research program at Cambridge Hospital, and S. Nassir Ghaemi, MD, director of the bipolar disorder research program at Cambridge Hospital and assistant professor of psychiatry at Harvard Medical School. The BSDS is a self-report form. The BSDS was designed to help diagnose people who present with subtle symptoms of bipolar disorder. The BSDS, based on specificity and sensitivity, is useful as an adjunct in the diagnosis of bipolar disorder, especially bipolar II (Nassir Ghaemi, Miller, Berv, Klugman, Rosenquist, & Pies, 2005) (BSDS is found online at www.psycheducation.org/depression/BSDS.html.)

Screening for Obsessive Compulsive Disorder

Any health care provider involved with the care of women during the postpartum experience should actively screen for symptoms, especially in the early weeks. It is the simple question that needs to be asked: "It is not uncommon for new mothers to experience intrusive, unwanted thoughts that they might harm their baby. Have any such thoughts occurred to you?" (Brandes et al., 2004). If the response is positive, the Yale-Brown Obsessive Compulsive Scale (Y-BOCS) is an easy to administer scale (Goodman et al., 1989a). It may also be useful to ascertain treatment responses at subsequent visits.

The Y-BOCS is a clinician rated scale made up of 10 items. Each item is rated from 0 (no symptoms) to 4 (extreme symptoms). The total score can range from 0 to 40, with separate subtotals for severity of obsessions and compulsions. Interrater reliability for two psychiatrists for the total Y-BOCS scores was r = 0.98 (Goodman et al., 1989a). Internal consistency reliability was reported as r = 0.89. With a sample of 81 obsessive compulsive disorder patients, convergent validity of the Y-BOCS was demonstrated with the Clinical Global Impression-Obsessive Compulsive Scale (r = 0.74) and with the National Institutes of Mental Health-Global Obsessive Compulsive Scale (r = 0.67) (Goodman et al., 1989b).

References

American Psychological Association. (2000). *Diagnostic and statistical manual of mental disorders* (4th ed., text revision). Washington, DC: Author.

Beck, C. T. (1992). The lived experience of postpartum depression: A phenomenological study. *Nursing research*, 41, 166–170.

Beck, C. T. (1993). Teetering of the edge: A substantive theory of postpartum depression. *Nursing Research*, 42, 42–48.

Beck, C. T. (1996). Postpartum depressed mothers' experiences interacting with their children. *Nursing Research*, 45, 98–104.

Beck, C. T. (2001). Predictors of postpartum depression: An update. *Nursing Research*, 50, 275–285.

Beck, C. T. (2002). Revision of the Postpartum Depression Predictors Inventory. *Journal of Obstetric, Gynecologic, and Neonatal Nursing*, 31, 394–402.

Beck, C. T. (2003). Recognizing and screening for postpartum depression in mothers of NICU infants. *Advances in Neonatal Care*, 3, 37–46.

Beck, C. T., & Gable, R. K. (2000). Postpartum Depression Screening Scale: Development and psychometric testing. *Nursing Research*, 49, 98–104.

Beck, C. T., & Gable, R. K. (2001). Further validation of the Postpartum Depression Screening Scale. *Nursing Research*, 50, 155–164.

Beck, C. T., & Gable, R. K. (2002). *Postpartum Depression Screening Scale Manual.* Los Angeles: Western Psychological Services.

Brandes, M. Soares, C.N. & Cohen, L.S. (2004). Postpartum onset obsessive-compulsive disorder: Diagnosis and management. *Archives of Women's Mental Health*, 7, 99-110.

Cox, J. L., Holden, J. M., & Sagovsky, R. (1987). Detection of postpartum depression. Development of the 10-item Edinburgh Postnatal Depression Scale. *British Journal of Psychiatry*, 150, 782–786.

DeMier, R. L. (1994). Predictors of posttraumatic stress disorder in mothers of high-risk infants. Unpublished doctoral dissertation. University of Wisconsin-Milwaukee.

DeMier, R. L., Hynan, M. T., Harris, H. B., & Manniello, R. L. (1996). Perinatal stressors as predictors of symptoms of post-traumatic stress in mothers of infants at high risk. *Journal of Perinatology*, 16, 276-280.

Dennis, C. L. (2004). Influence of depressive symptomatology on maternal health service utilization and general health. *Archives of Women's Mental Health*, online, June 15, 2004.

Driscoll, J. (1990). Maternal parenthood and the grief process. *Journal of Perinatal and Neonatal Nursing*, 4, 1–10.

England, S. J., Ballard, C., & George, S. (1994). Chronicity in postnatal depression. *European Journal of Psychiatry*, 8, 93–96.

First, M. B., Spitzer, R. L., Gibbon, M., & Williams, J. B. (1997). *User's guide for the structural clinical interview for* DSM-IV *axis 1 disorders*. Washington, DC: American Psychiatric Press.

Goodman, W. K., Price, L. H., Rasmussen, S. A., Mazure, C., Fleischmann, R. L.Hill, C. L., Heninger, G. R., & Charney, D. S. (1989a). The Yale-Brown Obsessive Compulsive Scale I: Development, use and reliability. *Archives of General Psychiatry, 46*, 1006–1011.

Goodman, W. K., Price, L. H., Rasmussen, S. A., Mazure, C., Delgado, P., Heninger, G. R. & Charney, D. S. (1989b). The Yale-Brown Obsessive Compulsive Scale II: Validity. *Archives of General Psychiatry, 46*, 1012–1016.

Gruen, D. (1990). Postpartum depression: A debilitating yet often unassessed problem. *Health and Social Work, 15*, 261–270.

Harberger, P., Berchtold, N., & Honikman, J. (1992). Cries for help. In J. A. Hamilton & P. N. Harberger (Eds.), *Postpartum psychiatric illness: A picture puzzle* (pp. 41–60). Philadelphia: University of Pennsylvania Press.

Harkness, G. (1995). *Epidemiology in nursing practice*. St. Louis: Mosby.

Hearn, G., Iliff, A., Jones, I., Kirby, A., Ormiston, P., Parr, P., et al. (1998). Postnatal depression in the community. *British Journal of General Practice, 48*, 1064–1066.

Heneghan, A. M., Mercer, M., & DeLeone, N. L. (2004). Will mothers discuss parenting stress and depressive symptoms with their child's pediatrician? *Pediatrics, 113*, 460–467.

Hirschfeld, R. M. (2002). The Mood Disorder Questionnaire: A simple, patient-rated screening instrument for bipolar disorder. *Primary Care Companion Journal of Clinical Psychiatry, 4*, 9-11.

Holopainen, D. (2001). The experience of seeking help for postnatal depression. *Australian Journal of Advanced Nursing, 19*, 39–44.

Huysman, A. M. (1998). *A mother's tears*. New York: Seven Stories Press.

Kennerley, H., & Gath, D. (1989). Maternity Blues I: Detection and measurement by questionnaire. *British Journal of Psychiatry, 155*, 356–362.

Kleiman, K. R., & Raskin, V. D. (1994). *This isn't what I expected: Postpartum depression*. New York: Bantam Books.

Lawrie, T. A., Hofmeyr, G. J., de Jager, M., & Berk, M. (1998). Validation of the Edinburgh Postnatal Depression Scale on a cohort of South African women. *South African Medical Journal, 88*, 1340–1344.

MacLennan, A., Wilson, D., & Taylor, A. (1996). The self-reported prevalence of postnatal depression. *Australian and New Zealand Journal of Obstetric and Gynecology, 36*, 313.

Murray, L., & Carothers, A. D. (1990). The validation of the Edinburgh Postnatal Depression Scale on a community sample. *British Journal of Psychiatry, 157*, 288–290.

Nassir Ghaemi, S., Miller, C. J., Berv, D. A., Klugman, J., Rosenquist, K. J., & Pies, R. V. (2005). Sensitivity and specificity of a new bipolar spectrum diagnostic scale. *Journal of Affective Disorders, 84*, 273–277.

Stein, G. (1980). The pattern of mental change and body weight change in the first postpartum week. *Journal of Psychosomatic Research, 24,* 165–171.

Thompson, W. M., Harris, B., Lazarus, J., & Richards, C. (1998). A comparison of the performance of rating scales used in the diagnosis of postnatal depression. *Acta Psychiatrica Scandinavica, 98,* 224–227.

Thome, M. (2003). Severe postpartum distress in Icelandic mothers with difficult infants: A follow-up study on their health care. *Scandinavian Journal of Caring Science, 17,* 104–112.

Wiley, C. C., Burke, G. S., Gill, P. A., & Law, N. E. (2004). Pediatricians' views of postpartum depression: A self-administered survey. *Archives of Women's Mental Health,* online, July 19, 2004.

Zelkowitz, P., & Millet, T. H. (1995). Screening for post-partum depression in a community sample. *Canadian Journal of Psychiatry, Revue Canadienne de Psychiatrie, 40,* 80–86.

APPENDIX

MEDICATIONS: PREGNANCY AND LACTATION

MEDICATIONS	FDA CLASS USE IN PREGNANCY[1]	RELATIVE SAFETY IN USE WITH BREASTFEEDING
Anxiolytics and Sedatives		
• Alprazolam (Xanex)	D	Little data available; if used, minimize dose and duration of use (Hendrick & Gitlin, 2004)
• Buspirone (Buspar)	B	
• Clonazepam (Klonopin)	D	
• Diazepam (Valium)	D	
• Flurazepam (Dalmane)	X	
• Lorazepam (Ativan)	D	
• Temazepam (Restoril)	X	
• Zolpidem (Ambien)	B	
Antidepressants		
• Amitriptyline (Elavil, Endep)	D	6 studies: appears relatively safe
• Bupropion (Wellbutrin)	B	1 study: no adverse infant effects
• Citalopram (Celexa, Lexapro)	C	3 studies: appears relatively safe
• Clomipramine (Anafranil)	C	3 studies: appears relatively safe

(continues)

Medications	FDA Class Use in Pregnancy[1]	Relative Safety in Use with Breastfeeding
• Desipramine (Norpramin, Pertofrane)	C	1 study: appears relatively safe
• Doxepin (Adapin, Sinequan)	C	3 studies: some adverse infant effects
• Duloxetine (Cymbalta)	C	No studies to date
• Fluoxetine (Prozac, Sarafem)	C	9 studies: some adverse infant effects
• Fluvoxamine (Luvox)	C	4 studies: appears relatively safe
• Imipramine (Tofranil)	C	3 studies: appears relatively safe
• Mirtazapine (Remeron)	C	No studies
• Nefazodone (Serzone)	C	1 study: adverse infant effects
• Nortriptyline (Aventyl, Pamelor)	D	6 studies: appears relatively safe
• Paroxetine (Paxil)	C	4 studies: appears relatively safe
• Sertraline (Zoloft)	C	7 studies: appears relatively safe
• Trazodone (Desyrel)	C	No studies
• Venlafaxine (Effexor)	C	2 studies: no adverse infant effects noted
Mood Stabilizers		
• Lithium (Lithobid, Eskalith)	D	Caution with use
• Valproate (Depakote, Depakene)	D D	Compatible (AAP)
• Carbamazepine (Tegretol)	C	Compatible (AAP)
• Fluoxetine/olanzapine (Symbyax)	C	No data
• Gabapentin (Neurontin)	C	No data
• Lamotrigine (Lamictal)	C	No data
• Oxcarbazepine (Trileptal)	C	No data

(continues)

Medications	FDA Class Use in Pregnancy[1]	Relative Safety in Use with Breastfeeding
Antipsychotics		
• Aripiprazole (Abilify)	C	Little known
• Clozapine (Clozaril)	B	
• Fluphenazine (Prolixin)	C	
• Haloperidol (Haldol)	C	
• Olanzapine (Zyprexa)	C	High doses have reported development delays in children
• Risperidone (Risperdal)	C	1 case report: no adverse effects
• Quetiapine (Seroquel)	C	1 case report: no adverse effects
• Trifluoperazine (Stelazine)	C	
• Ziprasidone (Geodon)	C	

[1]FDA Use in pregnancy ratings: (Physician's Desk Reference, 55th edition. Montvale, NJ: Medical Economics Company, 2001, p. 344).

    A: Controlled studies in women show no risk.

    B: Animal studies show no risk, but there are no controlled studies in humans, and animal studies show adverse effect that has not been confirmed in human studies.

    C: Animal studies show risk, but there are no controlled studies in humans. Studies in animals and humans are not available.

    D: There is evidence of risk in humans, but the drug may have benefits that outweigh the risk.

    X: Risk outweighs any benefit.

References

American Academy of Pediatrics. Committee on Drugs. (2001). The transfer of drugs and other chemicals into human milk. *Pediatrics, 108,* 776–789.

Ernst, C. L., & Goldberg, J. F. (2002). The reproductive safety profile of mood stabilizers, atypical antipsychotics and broad-spectrum psychotropics. *Journal of Clinical Psychiatry, 63*(Suppl 4), 42–55.

Gjerdingen, D. (2003). The effectiveness of various postpartum depression treatments and the impact of antidepressant drugs on nursing infants. *Journal of the American Board of Family Practice, 16,* 372–382.

Hendrick, V., & Gitlin, M. (2004). *Psychotropic drugs and women: Fast facts.* New York: W. W. Norton & Company.

INDEX

Note: f = figure
      t = table